UNCONSUMED

In His Abiding Grace

S.THUAM SIAM NGAIHTE

Unconsumed In His Abiding Grace

By S. Thuam Siam Ngaihte

©2019 S Thuam Siam Ngaihte
www.abidings.com

ISBN: 9781798781517

All Rights Reserved

For Ching Ngaihte, Mung Ngaihte, and Kim Ngaihte for their love and patience.

Contents

Introduction

Have you ever been through dark pits where no one could tread along? Well, we all did. Yet it has its different forms and phases. These phases of life show an unseen hand that holds us even when we didn't recognize it.

Every little or minute decisions, happenings, detours, unseen happenings of life, and the subsequent occurrences can either consumed us. On the other hand, if one remained unconsumed, it can shape our living.

Several times I woke up from being unconscious. Every time I woke up, the Lord is still with me. He let me live; so I'm alive because of his abiding grace.

Once when I woke up from seizure, I decided to pen down what I have seen. First, I am not a writer but in the hope of spreading hope and inspiring others, I wrote the words given to me in my broken state.

Life's adverse moments in pain and suffering, illness and financial breakdown, losing a job and the struggle of trying to be normal, are the blessing in disguise, which let me walk closer to God.

The word unconsumed has long been from the verse given to me in my times of despair: when alone with God in the small prayer cabin and in the fumigated room of Intensive Care Unit in the hospital. One can be weak and still remained unconsumed; emanating stronger, refined version, and weak but dependent on the Sovereign Lord.

Unconsumed simply means not consumed, not used up completely, or something remains. A thing or being going through something, which can consume them, but emerging safe or in the least still few useable qualities intact, is called unconsumed.

For instance, a metallic substance going through the refiner's fire, but not consumed by the fire, emerging stronger, shinier, and malleated into the desired shape is one example. Here, it should be noted that the metal was not consumed by the fire.

In other words, the art of not perishing despite circumstances unbearable to human being, only by the grace of God, is what I wanted to talk about here in this book.

For some readers, I understand, it might sound absurd to take shelter – holding onto the One we've never seen. Yet I urged you to please go through it and see for yourself.

When we're fully consumed, one day, we'd walk the stairs bridging heaven and earth if we stay loyal to the slain Son of God. But before that, I pray we fight the good fight till the very end. (1 Tim. 6:12)

It would be incomplete for me not to mention some people who are being with me. They are the face where I saw the abiding goodness of the Lord. Yet I can't mention all of them here personally.

I thank my wife Ching for her patience, encouragement, hard work, and being with me despite all the circumstances we faced. Also, my two little children Mung and Kim for their fervent prayer and faithful companion to me. Lastly to my father and brother, who prayed for me before he went to the Lord, and all my family and extended family members.

Chapter One

Imperfect People

Imperfect people are real people. Real people lived in the real world. And I am one of them. As long as we live in the real world, perfection cannot be attained; yet we must have hope, and for the best.

We grieved, suffered, heart-broken, pained, flawed, inferior, unfit, below standard, and felt incomplete. It is because we are imperfect people living in an imperfect world. It can consume us, it can shape us, and it can make our life worth living, as we remain unconsumed in the abiding grace of God.

People wanted to overcome our adverse moments with ease but somewhere down the line, our imperfection popped up. If and only, we're in our own strength, we're heading nowhere. The unseen work of God, behind the scene, only keeps us going.

It is natural that we have this longing for triumphing over this imperfection. We wanted to shine; be an example, leading a victorious life. In that pit of imperfection, we may fall, yet it can lead us to discover the meaning of life, should we rise again!

Imperfect Innate Being:

My father had taught me certain Christian values, which would keep my soul and body safe from the work of evil. I wanted to be a perfect boy at least by abiding with the rules of the house. Yet, sometimes, I ended up the opposite.

When I wanted to do good things, many times, I ended up doing what I hate. I want to live a life that pleases God and people around me. When we happen to make a hole in that imaginary boundary wall, we feel guilty.

Guilt-driven life has to be rescued with love. And many times I was rescued. But the thing is; the more you wanted to perfection, or at the least near perfection, our imperfection desire cropped up again. The saying, 'rules are made to be broken' holds true in young lives. And we have to fight the good fight, always!

Imperfect Body:

We possessed an imperfect body, which is susceptible to pain, developing wear and tear, as we age. Some become healthy while some battle for life since their very conception.

Several people had gone through the knives; developed a never-ending pain, scarred for life, and need consistent care. Yet some people had complete bones, organs, and hole-less skin, throughout their life. Still, they go through pain and hard times in some period of their life, which might be harsher than physical pain.

We are imperfect people waiting for perfection in the glory of the Lord. We are God's good work in progress. We eagerly await a Savior from there, the Lord Jesus Christ, who, by the power that enables him to bring everything under his control, will transform our lowly bodies so that they will be like his glorious body. (Philippians 3:20, 21)

Imperfect Character:

I have no skill for an interpersonal relationship with people. Handling relationships with persons near and far have always been an uphill task for me. But I am glad, there are enough people who still love me albeit my imperfections.

Decisions taken in our imperfect periods had led us to unwanted pitfall and hard times. Some are scarred for life, as our decisions followed by actions, once taken cannot be repealed. For many, it's just that tiny 'yes or no' moment, which bugged our life since.

My tongue is a small part of my body, which is the hardest to be tame. We can hurt someone without talking much; it is the quality of words we spoke than the quantity, which really matters. A small spark from our end can set a great forest on fire. (James 3:5, 6)

I may write about forgiveness yet I struggle to forgive others. It requires the work of the Holy Spirit. When somebody hurts us we wanted to bounce back. From our imperfect mind, there's hardly anything which is subtle and mild for others.

Some of us know the ways of getting closer to God but hardly act upon it. We are slow to make a decision when it matters most. Our acquired wisdom did not make us perfect rather it filled us with pride and self-esteem.

Hiding Imperfections:

We all tried to hide our imperfections. In this materialistic and unrighteous world, it is a good practice to conceal our imperfections, at some level. If not, we would have no respect and adore for people's personality or character.

Our ways of determining our imperfections are when: we don't have money, losing jobs, unemployed, unable to support our family, chronically ill, unable to maintain our status in the society, leading a lowly life, self-judgment, many more. And when our hide-out is no safer.

But we cannot conceal anything before the Lord, our Savior. We may lead a messy life yet God knows it all. Some of our lives are too messy that we might want to give up. However, our God accepts us, should we go to Him, despite our imperfections.

Trading Imperfections – On the Road to Perfection:

Some two thousand years ago, our Savior has flagged off a new bogie for us, towards the road to perfection. Since then, millions had boarded, some are on the road, while faithful and holy people had made it to perfection, in His abiding grace.

On the road to perfection, many get healed while some are made to wait for glorious revelation. We get delivered from our imperfections in His abiding grace; our sins and chronic illness gets washed by the atoning Blood of Christ.

In His act of Salvation, we are once again connected with Christ. Therefore, we have a hope of trading our imperfections as we headed towards becoming a perfect person in His abiding love. It is the greatest hope for imperfect people.

Our physical imperfections, appearances, scars, and adversities can be our stepping stone for building a strong and lasting bond of perfection with our Savior.

Christians are not perfect people, we have their imperfections too. But we are heading towards our road to perfection, in His abiding grace, when we humbled ourselves before our Savior.

On that day, when we met Him, we'd trade our imperfections with the complete perfections of our body and soul. We'd trade our sorrows and tears with joy and happiness. Our savior will wipe away our tears, which are shed because of our imperfections.

You First Loved Me

I still remember that feeling
That feeling deep in my heart
How can I forget the eagerness?
I am unable to hold any longer
I wanted to let it known to you.
When I realized, I have been loved.

You gave me Comfort
You gave me Hope
You gave me Love
Because you first loved me
Your son I had become
I love you, Jesus,
I love you Jesus, my Savior

Slained by my sinful soul,
Your sacrifice is overwhelming.
You rose from the dead
Victory o'er death you proclaimed
My wonderful friend forever be
In you, I will abide.

Chapter Two

Compassion & Hope: Renewed Every Morning

The same year I'd graduated from University, I had a seizure. To meet my immediate financial needs, I had started joining a private firm.

It was here, at my workplace, I'd suffered this unusual attack, which plagued my living since then. I was seized and my life-boat capsized. However, I just believe it was some jerking in my brain, which would soon vanish.

My preparations and night-long practices for my dream job had been hit hard. In some major competitive exams for jobs, I'd simply slept away my chances of getting jobs. Yet by God's grace, I secured a job in the banking sector, which I quit later.

In between work, I've been juggling and roaming through corridors of several hospitals in the hope of leading a smoother life but it wasn't meant to be, maybe, for the time being. Until several years ago, I'd started visiting the Intractable Clinics. I'd witnessed the moaning and giggling, in dereliction, of patients who encroached the corridors of the hospital.

Everything happens for a reason; reasons unknown or known, that I believe because I'd experience the other side of life too. Some of those very embarrassing moments are better left behind and forgotten. During the course of time, I was not consumed by my captivator, here seizure or epilepsy, it is because God's compassion failed not.

My family blueprint, which I'd developed through the years, could not be fully put into practice. The blueprint contained determined sources of income, administration, expressing love, tolerating each other, and holistic way of raising children, and the likes.

Through the struggles, life goes on. I went on to live a normal life, although illness persists, and get blessed in different ways. Sometimes, I termed it as an 'illness that comes too soon' mostly because I cannot see in God's view at this time.

There are times, in between, when it is difficult to find meaning in life. Yet I was not consumed by the work of evil inside my mind because the Compassion of Christ gets renewed every morning.

Although I don't want to admit it; enduring the pain and physical frailties throughout, was not easy. In the meantime, there are obligations and responsibilities, which can't ever be ignored.

His Compassions Fails Not:

I do believe that we all have verses in the Holy Bible, which renewed our hope in the face of adversity. When in financial deepwater and health-related issues, I was reminded of several verses. One of them is this:

Through the Lord's mercies, we are not consumed, Because His compassions fail not. They are new every morning; Great is Your faithfulness. (Lamentations 3:21-25) These verses have always comforted me and given me hope in times of adversities.

The Prophet Jeremiah had lamented during Jerusalem's captivity. Chapter 3 of the poem mostly dealt with his personal lamentation on the issue of suffering and God. The compassion of God brings hope to those who seek Him.

When in captives the people of Israelites lived a troubled life. Jeremiah the prophet had witnessed the unfathomable misery of God's people. The recent prosperity of Jerusalem has made their suffering all the more bitter. It is here in these verses a light of hope was shed again.

They are seized, held as captives by their enemies yet they are not consumed. The Lord was compassionate towards them. Again, let me reiterate here again that in their sufferings they are not consumed.

The Lord their God doesn't allow them to be fully consumed. Beyond their ability, they get protected. In the hope of returning one day, they still lived on. Through His prophet, he showed His compassion towards them in their sufferings.

My Renewed Hope Every Morning:

After several years of suffering, I'd undergo Brain Surgery two years ago. The aftermath has been filled with pain.

I'd developed migraines, which makes me, very much, sensitive to my surroundings and the pain was sometimes unable to bear. Being devoid of enjoyment in life is a huge challenge.

When I was rushed back to the hospital, it was not easy to endure the pain and shadowy images in my eyes. The day seems to be too long when you are suffering.

I waited for the night to come. I wanted to sleep. It is my hope that the morning would bring me something. Every morning my hope gets renewed.

In the midst of my physical frailties, it was good to have that feeling of hope. I still cherished that moment: when I am able to see the morning light. I'd prayed with huge hope of getting home soon.

All my wearies of yesterday are no more. The night has consumed my pain in the dark. A new morning has broken; a new hope has filled my heart. The love, mercies, grace, and compassion of the Lord were renewed every morning. It was a glad moment to rediscover I am still alive to see a new day. It is all because of the faithfulness of the Lord.

"The Lord is my portion," says my soul, "Therefore I hope in Him!" The Lord is good to those who wait for Him; to the soul who seeks Him."

In the face adversities, be it financial, health, relationships, His compassions fail not. The Lord gave me hope to carry on in this world. That hope, at some extent, made living with epilepsy easier. Hope becomes one of the most important pillars of my life.

Living in captivity: a life seized, was not easy. Yet I have this hope that deliverance is assured, and surely on the way.

It was more of a reminder to trust and put my faith in Him, so I weary not. It was a learning phase although it's difficult. The fruit would be sweet, one day, when the time comes. It is my hope that He would provide, fulfill, and gave us hope in times to come.

We will not be consumed in the process because His (God) compassion fails not! They are renewed every morning.

Chapter Three

Getting Ready

Before the time comes I wanted to get ready, if that's possible at all. But it happens most of the time before I could get ready.

I don't want to get embarrassed, amongst people, by these seizure attacks. When I have this aura, which warns me of the possible attack, I am very happy. Yet my happiness couldn't save me either.

Sometimes my SOS pill helped me avoid such circumstances. If it is going to happen; it happens. The most important thing is I wanted to finish my job or inform someone, in any case, I wouldn't recover.

If I'm out from home, there are times I'd call home to let them give a check on me every five to ten minutes. Nothing can be ascertained but anything can happen. If it's just another aura, then it's way better.

When I'm with my children alone at home, I'd tell them if something's wrong. My children would pray beside my bed, which gives me comfort. And God really did hear his prayer, which keeps me safe, most of the time.

When my God had cared and arranged help in my worst days, I am really grateful. He'd lead me home in those uncertain moments.

In my living with epilepsy, this is one of the many lessons it taught me. In any way possible, I could, I wanted to avoid unprecedented seizure attacks but one thing is inevitable, I could not stay safe all the time. Although there are some embarrassing moments, I was quite blessed enough, as I was saved from embarrassing moments.

Getting Ready for the End:

Talking about death is not always pessimistic. It can otherwise make us appreciate our lives, which inculcate optimism in our living.

Should we be clear about our beliefs; what we expect after death, it would help us in living a happy life. Each day of lives would be numbered. We'd give thanks to the Lord for the gift of time.

Let's get absorb in this matter and devote out whole time thinking about it. No, that is not my purpose of writing this. We should live as we could never die but get ready as we could die at any moment.

It might be clearer this way: It is hope, time and again here, that I'd awake again should I have seizure attack but with impending pain on my body. However, some episodes did change my analysis of my problem. Recovering, really, is not in my hand. Should it be time for me to go on there's nothing I could do about it.

The problem here is I could never be ready for such unprecedented episodes. But I have this faith that if something more than unusual happens in life, God took control of everything. The only thing I should be concern about is meeting Him again.

We shouldn't be left undecided about our future. One must be certain about our belief. If someone does not anticipate life after death or meeting our Savior, let's say it his choice now. But someone getting caught not readying for anything could be a disaster.

Apostle Paul, talking about the Day of the Lord, wrote to the Thessalonians: For you are fully aware that the day of the Lord will come like a thief in the night. (1 Thess. 5:2-11)

While citizens of every order are busy for (International, national, and local) "Peace and Safety" destruction will come suddenly on them. (My emphasis added) No one knows about the times and dates of such extent.

How do we get Ready?

Here in verses 8 to 11, the Apostle Paul gave a very brief yet meaningful instruction on getting ready so that no one should be surprised like a thief. Let's read:

"Putting on faith and love as a breastplate, and the hope of salvation as a helmet. For God did not appoint us to suffer wrath but to receive salvation through our Lord Jesus Christ. He died for us so that, whether we are awake or asleep, we may live together with him. Therefore, encourage one another and build each other up, just as in fact you are doing."

Salvation through the Lord Jesus Christ is the best way of getting ready being mentioned here.

For every beginning, there is an end. If a flower blooms today it will wither in few times. If someone is suffering there will be a time where suffering ends.

Some of the things in life are certain, that certainly we weren't interested. We are more drawn to those thrills of uncertainty.

In the meantime, let's work hard; not simply remain idle and disruptive. Let us help the weak, love each other in brotherly and sisterly love, and be patient with one another. (Verses 12-14) Let us be thankful and optimistic each day of our lives.

Being prepared or getting ready will enhance our productivity, which will increase our appreciation of life. If not, we'd go empty-handed to our Worthy Savior.

Getting ready is the most appropriate thing we can do on our own; we don't need to involve others. There's no need for investing a huge amount of time and money but our own heart. It is more of a state of mind.

In his very own words, Jesus Christ had alerted the disciples about being getting ready or readiness at any hour. Here, let's read again:

You must be ready because the Son of Man will come at an hour you do not expect Him. (Matthew 24:44)

It becomes the least likely trend of many people who are too much anxious about this timing. Some people, in a very unfortunate way, ended up taking their own lives, which is against conforming to the will of God.

In the process of getting ready, we should not be too much anxious about God's timing. In His most appropriate timing, Jesus Christ came on earth to save us. And in His most appropriate timing, He would call us unto Him.

When we are young, healthy, busy in our own work, and with few difficulties in life we tend to think less of this important aspect of life. Still, it is a good thing, I would say because it shows we're happy.

However, some people still missed this aspect of life even in their worst situation. They are blinded, circumstances had blocked their view: their wisdom, their riches, their dilapidated life, could become their evil strongholds. But the abiding grace of God is always kind and nigh.

Let the grace of God be with us while we get ready for His Kingdom!

Chapter Four

My Personal Journey

It was just another normal day in winter. My body is still weak from the recent surgery but recovering well. As usual, with my son, we wake up early and go for a walk in the park on a wintry morning.

Soon we get back home, had our breakfast and began our day. Had just undergone Brain Surgery last month but it seems I am recovering well. So even a small time spent with my families is sweet and treasured. It was almost noon when I feel something was wrong with me. I told my wife to get help from neighbors and bring me to the hospital.

My wife called our neighbors. They rushed to our place but by the time they reached I remain unconscious. They brought me to a hospital, they told. However, as I remain unconscious I remember none of the ordeals.

My wife told that they brought me first to Safdarjung Hospital – one of the largest Public Hospital in New Delhi, which is about 10 kilometers approx. from our residence. On being there, I was given some quick medication and was given oxygen through a mask.

But then, they had to rush me again to Govind Ballabh Pant Hospital – also a state-run hospital, which was about 11-12 kilometers from there. Govind Ballabh Pant Hospital was where I was operated on 14th December 2016. On being there, let's make it short, I recovered in the Emergency Ward.

But as for me, when I regained consciousness, I found myself waking up in the Intensive Care Unit, as they already shift me there. All through the ambulance journeys, from our residence and my short stay at Safdarjung Hospital to GB Pant Hospital, I knew or felt nothing as I was unconscious.

These are my recollections base on what they told me: During those hard and unconscious times, I knew I was there somewhere else, which was totally a different scene. I was there in the middle of the sky, up from the earth.

There I saw a huge and brightly lighted home that slowly moves towards me. By the time it came close to me, a gently slope stairway with around 10-12 stairs came down by my side. Then I saw a huge door, which was open for me.

Inside that huge door was a place filled with light. The kind of brightness in that light was different. It must be full of the Tree of Life.* It was soft and never seen before the light for me. That was a place of life. It seems to be full of oxygen. I very much wanted to go inside that door.

There is this feeling that when I entered that door, I would start dancing and be "very much alive" there. This is the place where there would be no more death. My sickness would disappear. Everyone would jump and dance in joy, this is how I felt.

The light, brightness, and the look of the place I find it hard to describe. I don't even know what to compare it with. With great excitement, I put my left leg to go up the stairway. At that moment, I heard someone calling me from a very far off distance. I could barely hear her voice. But I recognized the voice was my wife's.

Though I saw no one from that huge door, it seems someone is there and watching me. I said, "Lord my wife and my children are still there. They will need me." So I turn back to find her. But then, when I look down, I saw her deep down there on earth.

They are very far from me. She looks very sad as I can feel her for a moment. She was there sitting in great distress. But it was dark around her and the place was filled with black dirt in comparison with what was before me. That was when I felt I am back. All of a sudden, I knew that door and stairway are no longer there.

That was the last thing I knew. Back at the Hospital, my body was in severe pain when I regain my consciousness.

I longed for that place where I had almost been but to no avail. Many times I would say to myself, had I entered that door I would be very much alive and well. But now I have to fight the pain on my body again. However, all sickness and the pain were worth it as I catch a Glimpse of Heaven. During this episode, I was there inside the Ambulance or either in the Hospital fighting for my life.

In other words, it all happened when I was a shift to different places in an ambulance or in a trolley. But then I thank God to see the light of another day here with my family. Though it takes many days to recover from that, I am happy.

That is a reminder of where we would be after we are done with our life here on earth. Now my father and my brother must be there spending time with our Savior. In medical term, I underwent right Amygdalohippocampectomy 14th December 2015 to help cure my epileptic disorder, which I was fighting for more than nine years.

On 19th January 2016, an episode of Status Epilepticus occurred, that lasted for so long. I felt blessed and obliged to share this. Also, I feel humbled; to have a glimpse of Heaven.

All the prayers held for me are my lifeline now. I am happy to be alive to tell this to you. More importantly, I feel blessed to be accepted as a citizen in the kingdom of God by the blood of Jesus Christ. God bless you!

The Tree of Life:

After he drove the man (Adam for his sin) out, he placed on the east side of the Garden of Eden cherubim and a flaming sword flashing back and forth to guard the way to the tree of life. (Genesis 3:24)

On each side of the river stood the tree of life, bearing twelve crops of fruit, yielding its fruit every month. And the leaves of the tree are for the healing of the nations. (Revelation 22:2)

Amygdalohippocampectomy: removing the amygdala, a surgical procedure and Status epilepticus is a dangerous life-threatening condition in which epileptic fits follow one another without recovery of consciousness between them.

Chapter Five

Faithful and Merciful

It was not the first time for me to run into deep waters of life. Several times before I have taken a detour from the trajectory of life; sometimes as a result of personal failure and another time the reasons not known before or after.

January 21 reminded me of one such incident which could have been the end of me on earth. Please refer to my previous posts should you like to read about it.

However, when the valley of the shadows of death becomes the place where you spent more time with the faithful, in his mercy, it becomes the time you'd never forget. Not forget because it was too hard but because you can feel you are in the hand of someone whom you so trusted.

The joy and happiness coming out of my suffering I had already put it out here so many times. And I will do more, by the grace of God. The suffering and the pain at the time, or at that time, are unbearable but if that's the way to feel the compassionate love of God, it is still worth it.

Some people, right after reading or hearing what I have to say told me, they wanted to feel it that way. But it's a privilege to be in pain yet see the faithful God. The Lord is faithful, and that's what he is.

The Bible tells us in 2 Timothy 2:13, "If we are faithless, He remains faithful, for He cannot deny Himself."

I'm no faithful follower of Christ yet he is so faithful. Yet I dared to be called the follower of him in his grace. He is so merciful that a chance upon chance is being given upon us. It is worth telling.

Not Consume in His Mercy:

The bible verse, Lamentation 3: 22-25, speaks to my mind in my times of trouble. "Through the Lord's mercies, we are not consumed, Because His compassions fails not. They are new every morning; Great is Your faithfulness."

When we hit a roadblock in our life, we tend to retrospect. In my retrospection and inspecting the past, I have found myself to be unworthy of the care and love of God. My actions and decisions are demeaning for him and diminish his name among friends and family.

As you too might be, I know myself, and I know I am simply good to let it be consumed by the happenings of life. But in his mercy, only in his mercy, I am not consumed. I do not consume to see more of the faithfulness of him.

Not only we don't consume but we can have full hope in Him. And his righteousness fails not. His love and mercy endure forever.

With the Faithful Owner:

Let me insert herewith very short instances of my days tending to our water buffaloes. There are times when one among the herds got stuck in the mudslide after months of incessant rain in the region.

As the soil below the surface had loosened it is hard for the animal to climb out of the mud pit. At dusk when we counted and found our water buffalo missing we began our search operation. Once located, we toiled hard until we rescued the animal.

Sometimes we call for help as we need to dig a way out for the heavy animal. As the owner, we don't want them t be consumed by the natural disaster to the extent we could. This just the act of ours as the owner.

In that way, the good shepherd did not want any of us to perish in the way once and before we accepted him as our Savior. How comforting are these words: Jesus Christ said, "I am the good shepherd; I know my sheep and my sheep know me— just as the Father knows me and I know the Father—and I lay down my life for the sheep. (John 10:14-15).

Walking with the Faithful One:

Coming back to that day where I was rushed to ER, how my God had assembled help in the form of neighbors, relatives, and loved ones will be tales to tell. The smooth ride by ambulance, let me called it smooth since I remember none, as I was unconscious throughout, which was really smooth, was a true cause in handling and saving one's life.

We walked with God in our everyday life but his faithfulness being shown while we're in the valley of the shadow of death was more heartwarming. It gives hope sending out and within the positive atmosphere at a go.

In his mercy, our time through the valley had been turned into a spring of water, which will nourish the mind throughout our here on earth. So, let us take courage and have hope in the Lord.

Faithful and Protective:

Fear is something that is hard to defeat as it normally cropped up from our mind. The evil one, in ways we can't easily understand, tries sowing the seed of fear in our mind. And we did really fear our lives, although we may not confess anytime and anywhere.

In his faithfulness, our God is protective of the works of the evil should we seek help from him. The apostle Paul wrote to the Thessalonians as: "The Lord is faithful, and he will strengthen you and protect you from the evil one." (2 Thess. 3:3)

The Lord will protect us in our pilgrimage, here on earth, and will lead us home to him when the day for us had come. The promises of being with him, those who are saved, was re-affirmed here, to those who have hope in him:

"Let us hold fast the confession of our hope without wavering, for he who promised is faithful." (Heb. 10:23)

In the end, I (we) have been thrown down before but the faithful Lord pulled me (us) up again because the Lord is merciful.

Give thanks to the Lord
For he is faithful
Give thanks to the Lord
For he is merciful
His love endures forever.

Chapter Six

Hiding Tears

Hiding tears isn't easy; it can be agonizingly painful. Tears are an outcome of intense emotional strain caused by a certain level of happiness or an adverse effect of despair. Tears, once shed, can't be undone.

One day and as usual, I visited the hospital to get my forty minutes video-electroencephalography done. As I get there, I was informed that my time slot gets change, so I had to wait for another two hours. So I reclined myself into the waiting room and read several verses of the Bible from my phone.

Several minutes passed by when a young lady entered the waiting with pieces of cotton still reeling in her hair. She dropped her body down in the corner chair. Before long, I could sense her whimpering in reclusive, hiding in the shade of her torn tresses.

She was holding her tear; trying to hide it as much as she could, and she looked tired. So I enquired a little and asked her to let it out, to let her tears flow freely, in the hope that she'd get relived. Hiding tears is hard and it can be tormenting.

The young lady told me that she had the possibility of undergoing brain surgery, which she feared the most. In her words, her long-due sufferings of epileptic disorder gave her no chance to live her dreams.

For instance, her dream of meeting her prince charming get shattered and the attacks came in the least expected time. In a way, I feel blessed to be in that place so that she could let her tears out. Since

I have the same illness and underwent brain surgery, I try to comfort her in the best possible way I could.

However, there's some gap as we're of different faith and religion. As we're fighting the same disorder, I share her some life hacks: Finding the strength to go on with epilepsy at bay. How God gave me a life and beautiful family, despite in this condition. She told me that sometimes she simply cried in a secluded place because of her fate.

Like many, she became that random person, who we met for a short span of time, with a heavy heart and we wanted to help. Yet in a moment or two, she's gone with her attendant holding her now. Before she left the room I assured her I'd pray for her and I really did, that day.

When my time slot came, I went in, waited for the technician to put in the electrodes in my scalp. I doze off easily until my video electroencephalography is over, as they read my brain activity. It made me feel grateful to have supporting people with me throughout my suffering, unlike some sick people, gifted by God for my comfort and care.

Tears before God:

We all have tears; by letting it out it eases our suffering or pain. In moments of a higher degree of happiness and comfort, we still shed our tears. Most people hide their tears, as it can be misleading at times. It is taken as a sign of weakness in many forms.

No one wants to look sad; we wanted to appear happy and spread happiness in the best possible way we could. Yet we are reduced to tears in our most private moments. It is a result of our innate being. We are blessed to have tears, which can flow. It shouldn't be hidden.

Shedding tears before the Lord our God is by far the most appropriate place. Our God keeps counts of our tossing, and put our tears in His bottle. (Psalms 56:8) Our teardrops don't go in vain.

In my long years of suffering, I too shed tears yet I tried to hide as much as I could. The upside is that some of the tears are tears of joy in the midst of suffering. God sees our tears; this makes my sufferings easier though it didn't take away the pain.

Tears in Secluded Place:

When I'm full of bitterness, emotional strain, and wanted to let it out, I moved into a secluded place to weep before the Lord who is the creator of heaven and earth. Sometimes my secluded place can be in the woods (when I'm in the countryside), in the prayer cabins, and the corner of the church.

We are highly privileged to commune with God everywhere, even in our most appropriate or inappropriate timing and place. Appropriate, when we seek our own comfort and place; inappropriate, when we are in the middle of trouble and crowded places. Those tears before the Lord never go in vain, let me reiterated.

It is my belief that no one can tell our pain exactly as it happens. So we tend to hide most the pain inside as well as our tears. And we wanted no one to be intrusive in our life except for some designated or very close persons.

Still, there are some who never let their adverse moments known. It might be because it was taken as the quality of manliness. In a secluded place, no one bothers nor disturbs us, yet God sees us. We can openly let our tears flow crushing the pain of hiding tears.

When the tears run dry, sometimes immediately or very lately, the infilling and comfort of the Holy Spirit takes place. Although the waiting period may differ those tears becomes our treasured possession, which makes me move forward.

Man of Tears:

King David, in the Holy Bible, was a Man of Tears. Many instances are given indicating David wept loudly. He wept for God's people, for committing a sin, and many times because of the adverse situations in his life. Yet he had unfailing hope in the Lord.

For instance, when David and his men found the Amalekites had destroyed Ziklag they wept aloud until they have no strength left to weep. What a sorrowful event recorded in the Bible! Simply the thought of it still haunts me.

But David found strength in the Lord His God, it was recorded. In this time of distress, he turns to the Lord. In short, David and his men run after their enemies, overtake them, and destroyed them recapturing their possessions. (1 Samuel 30)

Tears can be our connecting link with our God thereby regaining our lost strength for our life and mission to carry on. David was a man who openly shed tears before the Lord his God. He said: "My tears have been my food day and night." (Psalms 42)

Many of the Psalms were a cry for help in the most devastating period of his life. He knows that God is his only possession, his rock, and salvation. His salvation comes from the Lord.

By opening himself with tears in his eyes, David had the privilege of being closer to the Lord while on earth. Let him be our source of inspiration in our dark days.

Trading Our Leaky Eyes:

In grieving, suffering, and non-anticipated hardship we easily shed our tears. When our life's underperforming, unable to keep up with peer pressure, and our life's boat developed leakage it is difficult to continue living joyfully.

When all our innate and acquired wisdom cannot set us free, unable to find alternatives to some living condition, it pains our heart. That pain caused tears to flow behind our eyelid and when it is more painful to hide that tears, remember you are not alone. There must be a purpose for that pain.

In those moments, it is better to turn to God and shed our tears before our Savior. Either way, our Savior lifts our heavy heart or gives us the ability and strength to endure that adverse period whether long or short.

Our God works for our own good; He's not selfish and zealous of our happiness and wellbeing. The same way the Holy Spirit helps us, He intercedes for us with wordless groans. The Spirit intercedes for God's people in accordance with the will of God. (Romans 8:26, 27) Let's put our leaky eyes before the Lord; Pour out our soul before our Savior. And if it is for His glory, our God will make us whole again.

> Tears roll down from my eyes
> Down in my cheek, it flows wide
> Put my tears in your bottle
> List my tears on your scroll
> For long I've been a sojourner

Hiding my tears agonizes me

See my tears, Lord!
Trade my tears with joy
Let my tears be a gel of happiness
Let my tears be the fragrance of my devotion;
Blossoming into glad songs as the 'Lark's
Spreading hope in gaiety's cheer.

Chapter Seven

The Waiting Period

"Don't be afraid. Jesus (Christ) will calm the storm when the time comes!" My five-year-old son consoled his baby-sister.

One evening, strong tropical monsoon winds blew the neighborhood unexpectedly. As it generally happened with our young ones, our little daughter was covered in fear. The trees bending up and down were a rare sight for her.

Few days before, I was narrating when Jesus Christ calmed the squall in the Sea of Galilee. The disciples were unhappy with their Teacher being asleep in such a dangerous situation. They felt He didn't care enough for them as they had expected. (Matt. 8:23-26)

No one knows know long the wind will blow. Nor did we have authority over the winds. Several measures can only be taken to take shelter. Modern technologies also failed to measure the exact consequences.

So, it is important to know what to do, how to do, just before 'the time' comes. Jesus Christ rose from the dead but after three days. The waiting period was three days.

On the road to Emmaus; "…we were hoping that it was He who was going to redeem Israel. Indeed, besides all this, today is the third day since these things happened." They are lonely and deeply troubled. The news of Christ's Resurrection, simply, astonished them. (Luke 24:19-35)

Several times, the pain, caused by the neurological disorder, in my body was hard to tolerate. Yet the time has not come when I will be completely free from it. It will come sooner or later, in His time.

So, in the meantime, I should not be left discourage or afraid. I needed to remind myself this more often than before. He will calm the storm one day.

Fear often overshadows faith. When the pain is there, it is a good reminder that I am conscious and fully alive. Fear kept the going troubled.

It is wonderful how one get strength - from where and when. This time it comes from my son. As he consoled his baby sister who was in distress, often times I am the one who needed to be consoled.

When you are hit back by what you've told others about comfort, being God as our refuge. It makes me wonder whether I did less in the past or not. It can become an important step forward in the way of life.

When God Says NO:

Here it is noteworthy that we do NOT get saved because of our own good will or work. We are not consumed because the compassion and grace fails not. It is only through the grace of God we become His children.

We cannot bargain with God because of our work. God is an entity which cannot be questioned; God is the supreme authority. And God, sometimes, says no to the request of His servants.

Moses, in his early life, traded his prestigious living advantage in the house of the Pharaohs for the love of his own people – the Hebrews. Moreover, he became the channel and staff of God in leading out the Israelites from captivity.

He suffered with them in the wilderness; lead the grumbling Israelites for years although with God-given authority. The service rendered by Moses to God through his servanthood was more than significant and notable. However, instances from the 'Water from the Rock' moments can't be nullified in the eyes of God.

Moses was forbidden to cross the river Jordan. He pleaded with God to let him see beyond the Jordan – the Promised Land – for which he has struggled with the Israelites. The Lord told him, "That is enough. Do not speak to me anymore about this matter." In other words, it is the Lord saying NO. (Deut. 3:21-29)

A few weeks ago, when a friend shared us these verses I found it to be very disturbing and disheartening. But it makes me believe more in the superiority of the Lord. He is the Lord, our God through Jesus Christ, who holds the future and knows what is best for His children!

It would be heart-wrenching the Lord saying NO to our pleadings and this never would be our anticipated reply. But Moses respected the decision of the Lord and he simply did not give up, at that very instance! Still, he lived for the Lord till he passed on the baton to Joshua.

Moses goes on to fulfill the remaining work required of him by the Lord, for His people. Do we simply turn away when we don't get what we pleaded for? Take some time out to think for yourself….. What is our reaction in those situations?

From this we know that Moses was a true and faithful man of God; he understands how the Almighty works. This is how the true men of God act and reacts.

In the end, the silent moment of God in our lives can lead us closer to Him. A NO to us from God can be a turning point in the mission of God, which further strengthen the lives of others. Sometimes we also say NO or nothing to our children for good.

The Lord does seem to remain silent at times, yet God simply did not forsake or abandon His Children forever!

Chapter Eight

Selfishness In Sufferings

There is no exception to our selfish ambition while in sufferings. Selfishness needs to be tamed, before it consumes us, although that's the hard part.

Selfishness resulted in suffering. And it is true the other way round. They go hand in hand yet they should not be together as selfishness would cause greater sufferings.

Here we will talk about selfish ambitions only in the context of a suffering person. Let us put aside those selfish ambitions for riches and personal gains for the time being.

Well, infighting has been going, on and on, in a suffering mind. It is caused by outward physical pain and daily happenings. In the end, selfishness becomes an integral part of a sufferer.

Entertainment, once they are, in the form of plays, music, and the likes, could become a hindrance in living a normal life. I have been in this situation for some time, maybe it's hard to get over it when you have a chronic illness. I won't talk deep about it here but there are occurrences I have to endure in my epileptic disorder. And sometimes it's difficult to blend in with the normal surroundings.

The pain in our body was caused in many forms; not all forms can be avoided. But there are times when I thought some of the causes could be avoided. That is when my selfishness came up. Selfishness, in turn, gave way to more pain in the mind. And, that's my problem too.

In living life, there are obligations that cannot be ignored. I feel bad when I cannot conform to the demands of the people around me. I felt that I was selfish because I have to limit my activities.

In that way, the interests of the people around me were neglected. At times, I found myself to be egocentric and self-centered in approach because of my weak physical condition.

Maybe, that is why the Bible gave no exception to any circumstances when selfishness could be utilized in normal living. Selfishness destroys unity and steadfastness to God.

There's none who enjoy life for a longer period in solitary. Just for a short time, it might be enjoyable. I am not sure about that. We must learn to adjust to the interest of others. Submerging in our self-interest is being selfish.

Disturbances in life could be a blessing. If there's nothing to bother life would be dull. Eventually, loneliness would ruin and kill our life.

Selfishness as a Stronghold:

A stronghold is a fortress where one can take refuge and safely dwelled within the minimum threat. Here, in this case, it is that fort inside our human heart where the evil could safely thrive in.

Selfishness could be a stronghold for the evil to dwell if it is not destroyed from time to time. If left unattended the fortress might be difficult to get uprooted. One must focus on that every day should we wanted to be left unconsumed.

It has a parasitic character which would eventually eat up its host; here our life or character. It has to be crushed, one day at a time, with the help of the Holy Spirit.

No one can simply spin ourselves in a cocoon while we are on the march. We are to work together as a team in a family, society, and in the church. Yet we are tempted, in many forms, to be a little selfish, manage ourselves, and stay away from people.

Beyond Selfishness:

Now, let's see, in the Bible, what Apostle Paul wrote to the Philippians:

"Do nothing out of selfish ambition or vain conceit. Rather, in humility value others above yourselves, not looking to your own interests but each of you to the interests of the others." (Philippians 2:2-3) There's no exception given here.

People suffer, even the righteous suffer yet they become the source of their renewed strength from the Lord. When the Lord blessed our sufferings it can bring joy in our life.

There is a time for all - time to suffer, time to rest. It is my hope that this phase would be used by God to strengthen my faith.

We all suffer but in different ways. There are no great and small sufferings, the pain inflicted might cause the same destruction. But in the blood of Christ, we can be whole again.

Rejoice in every situation, says the Bible. In reality, it is really difficult but there must be a way out, I hope. Let us present our request to God, in prayer and petition, with thanksgiving. (Philippians 4:4-7)

In that way, the peace of God will transcend understanding while suffering. Further, God would safeguard our heart and mind, in Christ Jesus, through our journey.

There are still many people, saints and servant-hearted, who could help others despite their sufferings.

Dear reader, if you too are still in your suffering phase I empathize with you. It is my prayer God would guide us through this phase without causing further self-inflicting pain in the process.

Selfishness to Unselfish Worship:

In the realm of spiritual worship, we can't keep the light to ourselves. Telling it to others is a way of letting the light shine. If one is a true benefiter of the light of the world, they will keep on spreading it.

Let your light so shine before men, that they may see your good works, and glorify your Father in heaven. (Matthew 5:16)

When we are free from selfishness, we can give glory to the Lord. Our selfish ambitions in other realms of living will weigh us down till the time we confess before God. Now I know my intentions are worthless without you. Let our worship be of a selfless act, only to glorify you for what the Lord has done for us.

Create in me a clean heart, O Lord.
And renew a right spirit within me.
You, O Lord, who knows my heart,
If there's anything good left within me
Be magnified through me.

Chapter Nine

Someone Like Us

It's a thing of the past; I would like to say, but not yet. The time hasn't come yet; it must be near. With God, His grace will keep us alive. And that's how reassurance goes in the middle of suffering chronic illness.

So here, let's talk a bit of epilepsy and is epileptic. This chronic neurological disorder caused pain, burning sensation, seizures, mild to high degree depression, and anxiety, to say the least.

In this big-big world, many people like us irrespective of geographical locations, income-financial status, social strata, race, color, and many more, fights the disorder. The journey has been eventful, always, with the unforeseen twist and turns.

There's someone like us who's always fare better than we did. But there are tons of people who are like us or a little bit of needing more than we did.

In the countryside where I was hailing, medication was almost nonexistent in the nooks and corner of the hills. Many patients could have lead a better life if proper medications and care were available.

They still fight till the very end, endure the grueling pain, anxiety and depression, and almost outcast(?) as they can't join the normal proceedings of life. There's nothing to take pride in being epileptic with good or proper medication although the side effects of some medicines are hard to bear.

I remember the epileptic man fully distraught by his suffering scaling up the dusty street in winters, and muddy streets in summers with his big bamboo stick in hand. The stick was meant to help his torn-nerve while moving.

Now that I knew something about the disorder proper diagnosing and medication might have loosened their nerve a bit should they avail proper treatment? I feel for them, yet there's hardly anything I can do now.

One thing, although it pains me to say, was that I must be thankful for what I get at least. That the consistent medication, brain surgery, and the privileged of having someone, with good knowledge to take care of me.

What I wanted to convey here is that there are many people like us who suffered; bluntly, with less care, and with less knowledge. They are someone like us too.

Should reaching out would help; I wanted to reach out to you assuring 'you are not alone' in your fight. But I'm not sure this might help. However, please do not give up as yet!

The discussion forums in some sites often provide helpful information like the Epilepsy Foundation. Yet our weak mind, although I don't want to call it as weak, easily intertwined with the suffering of others. And in the process, sometimes disturbs our mind.

Now, there are many who are suffering but not the exact disorder. As we're still reeling in the suffering world, we should remind each other there's always someone like us.

Knowing Someone Like us:

On the flip side, knowing that there are people like us would make us live our lives responsibly. It should make us appreciate our life; what we get and what we don't. The attitude of gratitude should be sown in our hearts.

In many legs of my hospital and diagnostic center visits, I've seen so many people like me. There are people whose conditions are worse. While there are times we interact flaming up hopes for our future, there are times we don't feel like talking at all.

Trying to give hope to others in difficult times isn't easy. But we should give it a try. Telling them about our attitude towards suffering might help others if it's in the will of God.

Someone Who Become Like Us:

While mankind has been under the looming cloud of the Evil One, sufferings in all forms gushed the entire generation. Evil reign upon them; and it was difficult to stay connected to the Creator for a generation to generation.

The Son of God, humbling himself, came; becoming someone like us. We called him Jesus, someone, who treads the cursed soil – adorning and suffering just as we did.

Jesus Christ becomes someone like us that we might become the righteousness of God in him. (2 Cor. 5:21 NKJV)

Promises for Someone Like Us:

He wept, (John 11:35) as he saw the kind of suffering we faced, especially in the face of death, as the Evil One's reign over us.

He dined with us, he physically bears our pain with us, he saw our needs and many more. He's betrayed, he's heartbroken, forsaken by the Father as he took our sin to cross. He really is someone who became like us.

It doesn't end there. He promises us a life beyond our sufferings and pains!

For Someone Like Us:

For someone like us, what we can do best is upholding them as we pray. We may not possess a good heart, unselfish attitude, and spiritual maturity but we can pray. Just as Jesus did, (John 17)

"I do not pray that You should take them out of the world, but You should keep them from the evil one."

Today, we all have sufferings and difficulties; some escaped, some defeated, some are still fighting yet unconsumed in the abiding grace of God. Should we all pray for someone like us there wouldn't be people left untouched by the spirit of God.

Praying for someone like us:

One day the time will come where you and I can do the groundwork, in some way, for Christ. Although I'm still in my recovering process I do have hope in Him. If there's someone like me, we must pray for them.

At the same time, touching the world through our prayer, especially for someone like us, is what we can do best. It doesn't involve finances but our heart only with a good connection with God.

Praying for each other:

Dear reader, if you are one amongst someone like me, I'm praying for you. Our health issues, financial problems, diminishing identity, relationships, and all sorts of situations, which plagued our livings. I pray that God sees the desires of our heart.

We must uphold each other in our Thanksgiving and prayers; giving hope to each other.

Our afflictions are many, our problems are aplenty, but let's offered it to the Lord. The Lord will deal with it. And when the time comes or when we learned the much-needed lesson from our suffering, it will end.

Someone Like Us

For someone like me,
My escape door's clutching tight.
Someone's called my name,
I answered as I groaned in despair.
It's from Son of God;
You'll be freed; free men now!

God became someone like us;
Humbled with grace yet mighty.
Someone bearing our pain,
Someone I'd called a friend.
Someone to walk with;
Someone to cry on.
Someone, someone,
Who saves me for eternity!

Chapter Ten

Five Ways of Living

Here in this chapter, let's see some types of living we been through or we have seen.

Intoxicated Living

'The world's not as I expected,' skeptically mused a person, time and again. Although it is supposed to show humor, it has some truth. The world has intoxicated our living by the time our conscience is put to practice.

Our mind becomes intoxicated with wants, selfish ambitions, adjustments with immediate neighborhood, and so on. Physically, we have been a pain, suffered, and many more, as we live our daily life. These all are signs of us being alive, so it's a blessing.

As if these weren't enough, we have tons of ways to get intoxicated with. Intoxication took away our understanding and makes us unwise, at times. Our imperfect mind showed up when we speak or acts as fools in our intoxicated state. A sinful living is an intoxicated living.

Necessary Intoxication:

The other day, medical practitioners took some amount of my blood, as they need to determine what had intoxicated my living. The level of the drugs in my blood, which I had taken for a decade, had to be maintained at the so-called normal level.

49

Dosages of my medicines would increase if it's lower than the desired level; or lowered otherwise. My intoxicated blood becomes a boon for my normal living. My movements and activities, however, get more limited than before. Intoxication affects my life in some way.

Our body cells, neurons, and blood are designed by our Creator to accept and intermingle with outside particles for good. They secrete and excrete to keep our toxic level well balance to sustain our life. We are fearfully and wonderfully made, which need consistent yet limited care, only to the level we could.

Intoxicated by Pain:

Pain has become part of my normal life. As I said earlier, to be able to feel the pain is another blessing. It is a sign of me being normal and alive. Let me tell you that I have been in a situation beyond pain, being unconscious, and the experience is worse than pain.

We all suffered some kind of pain, in different ways. When our pain is too much it can blind our thinking, which suppressed our hope. It intoxicated our thoughts and living. Yet most pains are temporary or at least for a lifetime. Our search for suppressing pain can become dangerous.

In our intoxicated life, with pain and suffering, we search for an entity or someone who'll listen to our groaning, occasionally. What if I can tell all? It may somehow ease my occasional pain but it is hard to find a good listener. We can be boring, a chronic complainer, and negative mindset to others.

Pain does not subside by telling someone throughout so we all chose to keep quiet as much as possible. It's better to report our level of intoxication, by pain, to the Lord's.

Intoxicated by Misery:

Hannah was mistaken as a woman intoxicated by drinking wine when she poured out her deep misery before the Lord God. In reality, she was intoxicated by misery. She was severely provoked by her rival because she was barren; unable to bear a son for her husband. (1 Samuel 1)

She's a woman; I cannot say with certainty the level of her troubled heart. It'd be difficult to empathize her being provoked. Dear women, you'll know better. Her misery was beyond the love and understanding of her husband Elkanah.

Hannah was in bitterness of soul, and prayed to the Lord asking for a son, and wept in anguish until her voice was able to come out.

Hannah's Surrender and Hope:

Imagine should you be in Hannah's state of mind, it pained me. One night, my chest was choked, as I read it to my children. She was excessively intoxicated by her misery.

She did not care for what people would think. The priest Eli had observed only her lips were moving, as she spoke to the Lord in her heart. She vowed to give the child to the Lord, should the Lord grant her prayer. This lady was in huge distress and she surrenders herself fully to the Lord.

Hannah knew that her situation has come to the level which can be solved only by the intervention of the Almighty God. In her own conviction, she went to the Lord, because she has HOPE in Him.

Beyond Hannah's Misery:

She said, "May your servant find favor in your eyes." Then she went her way and ate something, and her face was no longer downcast.

There is an upside to her misery. Hannah's misery took her into the ministry of God. She participated in God's plan by bearing a ruler and priest for the Lord. Her contribution or role in God's ministry will be remembered as she did not shy away but approached the Lord.

It is a great relief to read the next chapter, which consists of her praise to the Lord. The Lord had granted Hannah's prayer, she bore a son, named him **Samuel**. Samuel was dedicated to the Lord; he grows onto become a priest who ruled and anointed the kings for Israelites.

Hannah's Prayer of Gratitude:

In Chapter 2, Hannah's prayer of thanksgiving was recorded. Her heart was filled with joy; for she witnessed the good deeds of the Lord. Her bitter life turns into a rejoicing life. She proclaimed: (1 Samuel 2: 2, 8, 9)

"There is no one holy like the Lord; there is no one besides you; there is o Rock like our God. For the foundations of the earth are the Lord's; on them, he has set the world. He will guard the feet of his faithful servants."

One day, or at least once in a while, we'd be set free from our intoxicated living, by the grace of God. Now, a rejoicing heart is a blessed heart. We should know how to be thankful and show our gratitude once we're set free. When the sun shines let us be thankful for the sun; and the sun doesn't shine let us be thankful for the shad we got!

How to Get Free from Intoxicated Living?

We have talked in length the details of God's work in Hannah's life. She was set free from her misery because she went to the Lord's presence. She knew her problem was beyond men can handle. A sinful living is an intoxicated living.

By hoping in the Lord, with great perseverance, we will be set free from our intoxicated living. The time will come for us to be free from all kinds of troubles the world can bestow upon us.

And for that, there's a way to know the truth. When we know the truth we can trust in Him. Today, how are you intoxicated? Let's abide in Jesus Christ. As Jesus Christ had declared, **"the truth shall set you free."** (John 8:32b)

I know it is hard to let a day pass when we're in the midst of our afflictions and sufferings. Yet we have hoped, amidst our intoxicated living, through Christ Jesus!

Unconsumed: Burning Living

The burning sensation, on the side of my head and face, was hard to deal with. Putting ice on the affected area does not help, as it does not burn outwardly. It was this well-designed aura that I had, due to my neurological disorder, which serves as a necessary warning in the wake of performing my daily routine.

Later on, I realized that it was a privilege having this burning sensation before the big thing arrived. I have the chance to get ready - either by taking pills or saying a prayer, reporting it to the Lord. Yet the severe burning sensations are hard to endure. When it already started it is better to gear up myself till it subsides.

Although I did not intend to describe in details here, as I did it to my doctors, it starts from one point and leaves at the tip of the hands or toes. It gripped, must have gripped, the cells around which it occurs or traveled. Sometimes I try looking myself at the mirror to check if it damages my skin; it did not, as it was not actually burning. And after my brain surgery, two years back, I got relieved a bit.

It was the might of God in the display; I was like burning yet unconsumed in the abiding grace of God. Not all burning feeling or thing did not necessarily end up in burning up the body or materials. If the mind and heart are still intact it's sufficient, and you can still talk to God or count the fire-left-outs.

Yet we're still human with senses and emotions. So, we react as we endure the burning moments, although in different ways. Some get angry at one time, while some complaint and others silently endure the phase. In the end, it is our state of mind which really matters; we can feel unconsumed in the abiding grace of God.

Literally, we're living a burning life; there are burned up parents, burning energy as we work hard, trying hard to burn unwanted calories, burning mind as we struggle to keep checks and balance, burning stack for recycling, temperature rising burning the ice-covered land, and many more.

Burned Yet Unconsumed:

In the burning thing, and/or experience we can see more of the might of God, as I said earlier. A well-trained yet runaway man met

God, in the wilderness of his life and place, through observing the burning bush. His name is Moses, the faithful servant of God.

Moses saw a flame of fire amidst a bush, in Mount Horeb, where he kept the flock of Jethro, his father in law. So he looked, and behold; the bush burned with fire, but the bush was not consumed. He turned aside to see why the bush does not burn.

When the Lord saw he turned aside, He called onto his name, directed to take off his sandals because where the Lord is; it is a holy place. Now the Lord gave Moses a life-long task of delivering His people from the oppression of Egypt till the Promised Land. (Exodus 3)

In very short, Moses give-in to be part of God's mission, which involved him walking and talking with the Lord as they lead the Israelites, throughout his lifetime. Trusting, putting on faith in the Lord, who burned yet unconsumed the bush, was a game-changer moment in the life of Moses.

Inside The Burning Fiery Furnace:

Now I want to take you the three young men who'd spent time with the son of God inside the burning fiery furnace. This was the decree of King Nebuchadnezzar:

At the sound of the horn, flute, harp, lyre, and psaltery in symphony with all kinds of music all people, under the command of the Babylonian king should fall down and worship the gold image the king himself had set up. And failing to worship the gold image would invite throwing them perpetrators in the burning fiery furnace, alive.

The three young men faithful to the living God – Shadrach, Meshach, and Abednego, however, did not worship the gold image which angered the king. Then they bound these men, in the king's order, and cast them into the midst of the burning fiery furnace.

Inside the burning fiery furnace, the king saw, four men, walking loose in the midst of the fire. They did not get hurt, and the fourth is like the Son of God. The three men were seen enjoying special time with their God, in the most unlikely situation of their life, inside the burning furnace. (Daniel 3)

They were burned yet unconsumed in the abiding grace of God. The harshest punishment molds them into a stronger warrior of God. Their burning experience thwarted the work of evil, turned their hostile situation into celebration proclaiming the work of God through their lives. The king, then instructed, all people to worship the God of the three faithful young men.

Beyond Our Burning Living:

It would be wrong to play with fire. But when the fire of evil tries burning our living, it would be wise to curb the fire before we get burned. We get burned in various ways and at different degrees. More importantly, we have a mighty God who restores the burned.

We have a fragile heart, which gets burned very easily. In today's world, we expected God to act on our behalf, work His way out and spare us of undesired burning. But in reality, that is not the case. There are times we need to experience the smell of burning so that we get more refined.

Some, as it seems to us, did not even go through the fire like Moses but saw the burning of the bush. Yet we cannot compare with the fate of others. They may not go through the fire, which is visible to the human, but they still have battles to battle in certain ways.

The refiner's fire is always burning, for you and me, to get refined. The sort of each one's work was revealed in the fire. If anyone's work is burned, he will suffer loss; but he himself will be saved, yet so as through fire. Yet it is hard to go through the burning period. (1 Cor. 3:15)

The more you get burned, the more you will get thirsty for more sweet little drops of water. We are cautioned many times in life; however, we still get burned in the unending lust and desires of the body and heart. (Romans 1:27)

Let me reiterate here and again that, in certain ways, I have lived the burning living, which is not the end of the world. When we called and acknowledge our desires to the Lord, as we went through the burning furnace of life, our God enjoyed being with us through the fire, while we waited for the king (as in the three young men's case) to take us out of the fire.

Our body may get burned, living through a series of burning experience, yet the soul will see the goodness of the Lord, most high. There are numerous elements and ways which could burn our heart, mind, and body. But, in the abiding grace and mercy of God, we are not consumed. (Lamentations 3:22-25) And, in the midst of my burning living, I thanked God for His abiding grace.

Privileged Living

Life is short, fragile, and mortal; yet it is a privilege bestowed upon us to live a life, just once. Some people enjoyed better living condition or status, making them appeared more privileged, while some people seem deterred by privilege. And it is true, privilege sans some people should they think so.

Privilege, by definition, is a special right and advantage, which was granted or available to a particular person or group. The privilege of a Christian is an exemption from the impending punishment due to our sin and having special rights to called God as our Father. (Galatians 4:6)

Ten decades ago, the Gospel of Christ shed light on our community. We have become subject to the Authority of God through His son, Jesus Christ. The deceiving and alluring power of Satan may knock down a few people but a certain number of people enjoyed living the privileged life under the authority of God. (Ephesians 1:21)

Now, do you really felt privilege, living under the authority of God, the authority of Jesus is far above all rule and authority and power and dominion? Is maintaining an abiding relationship with Jesus simply tiresome when you can perform part of the sacrifice by yourself? Let's leave it here for us to think and answer.

A number of times I have come across some people who do not find the need for one man to sacrifice for all mankind when they can offer burnt offerings and sacrifices on their own. The sacrifice of the Son of God for the atonement of our sins is abiding, should we put our faith and believe in His act of love, displayed on the Cross. For some, it is hard to trust one entity to work on them for nearing perfection.

But as for the believers, due to the great love the Father has lavished on us, I am one among the children of God. And that is what we are, our privilege! For the world who did not want to know Him, His act of love is in vain and foolishness. (1 John 3, 1 Cor. 1:25) It is not the question of affordability for sacrifices but the love which is shown. It is more about trusting on the Covenant, God made with mankind through His son, for this life and beyond.

Further, I agree that there are rituals we can perform on our own. However, it is beyond that. I don't know why you become a follower of Christ but it is a privilege living, riding on the sacrifice of Christ which liberated us.

We can love Him because He first loved us! I am privileged because Jesus loved me. Not only did He love; He saved me. Not only did He save; He cares for me! It is Jesus Privileged Me.

Privileged Companionship:

In sickness and in health, in poverty and riches, we have the privilege of walking with Jesus. Further still, when we cannot walk and slumber in insecurity, He sits and chats with us. The Lord is our refuge and our strength. It is safe being with Him. (Read Psalms 23 and 91 for more)

Waking up inside the walled Intensive Care Unit, the beeping sounds of life supporting machines grew loud and wild. My heart raced and the mind roamed, although with blurry memories, due to my unprecedented health failure and beyond. There in the wilderness, my privilege companionship with comfort the heart for a while.

As a pilgrim in progress, the compassion of Christ trimmed my loneliness and helplessness. It gave me a privilege of whispering to Him, sometimes in my choked voice, which gave hope in the temporary shelter of life. (Matthew 28:20b, Acts 16:25)

Privileged Suffering:

Suffering is and never was easy to endure. But with Christ, it becomes a school of learning the way of trusting more in His authority. There are many who graduated from the School of Suffering, where even the Biblical Job graduated. (Job 31) And it leads them to live a more privileged life than before.

Yet without Jesus, it's just a pain sans the privilege that simply deteriorated the body and soul. In the interim, we talked more, we think about God more often than we did in our normal life. In that way, it becomes the necessary evil which led us to discover more of the privilege we are bestowed in Christ.

As we headed for destruction or our mortality to take over our breath, we have the privilege of choosing the lighter yoke. The lighter yoke is being offered by Jesus to us the weary traveler. (Matthew 11:29) The more the questions we wanted to ask Him the closer we rallied to Him, in His abiding grace. In my suffering, it's a privilege being Him with me as it happened for a purpose.

Privileged Detours:

Nothing in the world is constant; it appears and disappears. Sad but true, our existence is also included. We plan a life; have a dream and on-course to achieving it. Just then detours, although not permanent, usually take over the wheel.

The Israelites are lost in the wilderness for forty years before stumping their feet on the Promised Land. Joseph's detours, in the pit and prison cell, before becoming the savior of his family during the famine, are necessary detours. It wouldn't be easy to endure treading real-time detours. (Genesis 37)

The most important to be noted here is that with Jesus Christ our adversities are no more constant. They are the necessary fluctuations of life. We have the privilege of having Jesus as our anchor, in these moments, so that we wouldn't get lost in the sea of life. It's a privilege as detours in life are not forever.

Privileged Rewards:

Our needs are rewarded through our simple prayers. The God, who feed the sparrows, without them sowing a single seed, is our God. In His abiding grace, our God rewarded each man and women according to our needs. (Matthew 10:29-32) It's a Jesus-Privileged-Me as I am under the authority of Him.

In our unlimited wants, however, we desire for more and never get content. Our loving God channelized our needs, and their sources, beyond the thought of our mind. Some work hard in the night, while we sleep peacefully so that we will be getting our daily necessities. In His authority, he commanded everything for the best of us.

Privileged Intercession:

We talked about the joy of having the liberty of talking to God, wherever and whenever, we wanted to. In reality, it is possible because we have the Holy Spirit, through the work of Christ, who intercedes for us.

The Spirit helps in our weaknesses. We do not know what we should pray for as we ought, but the Spirit Himself makes intercession for us with groaning which cannot be uttered, according to the will of God. (Romans 8:26-27) In our privilege living, we speak our mind to the Lord as we deemed fit. It's a Jesus-Privileged-Me because the Holy Spirit intercedes for me.

Unchanging Amount of Privilege:

The privilege we have in Jesus Christ is never-changing, as He never changes. Yesterday, today, and forever Jesus is the same. The love of God, poured out through His son Jesus Christ, never fluctuates. Nothing can deter us from our son-ship, once we abide in Him.

Every year Forbes richest lists are released. This year Jeff Bezos, from Amazon Inc., topped the ranking. In the next few days, the volatile market played its role, which makes him lose some million. Although he still retained his first position, further fluctuations in his market shares could prove detrimental.

However, in the case of enjoying the privilege of God's love, the love that comes from Him never fluctuates. If the love of God is anything like that can end or fluctuates depending on applied terms and conditions, it would reach me no more. Do you think, even without Jesus, your life or the fate of yours would be pretty much the same?

#Jesus-Privileged-Me:

Now the lists can go on and on. You can add more and inspire more. "The Lord is my portion," says my soul, "therefore, I hope in Him". And it's an unending privilege in everything not simply on the blessings or good part. A privileged living may fall yet it would rise again. (Psalms 119:57, Lamentations 3:24)

Looking back at my life, I have come across hurdles due to poverty, poor health, bad decisions, detours, some private failure which I don't want to disclose as yet, and many more. But through the love of Christ, I felt privileged to live a privileged life.

Do you really think it's a privilege knowing and following Christ, even when God doesn't make any sense? If so, let's start a campaign together using the hashtag, #Jesus-Privileged-Me, acknowledging our privileges to follow and chose Jesus.

Messy Living

It is easier creating a mess than untangling any kind of a mess. In our daily living, we messed with people either in a good or bad way. All kinds of messing are not bad; it depends on how we messed with and how often do we clean up our mess.

Believe it or not, the messed created by self have a far greater impact in our life as we have none to blame. Some of us are buried in our own mess which needs the rescue act of other people or entity. And for some, cleaning their own mess mold them grow into a stronger or successful person. Whatever the mess is; life must go on.

One day, for you to understand better, we were playing a board game with my children. Since it is a game of only two players, we couldn't accommodate our younger. Once we become more focused, we became quieter, which bored the on-looker. So, she protested by messing with us.

In a moment or two, we need to calm down the situation should we continue to carry on with the game. Although our game was halted briefly, it sends a message that needs to be taken care of. Thus it benefited all of us, as we spend the day further.

The problem, sometimes, is when we messed with people or people messed with us unintentionally. It is hard to understand what people go through in their life. And yet we messed with their living which many times add their load or devoid of their happiness.

Incidentally or accidentally, when our living becomes chaotic, tangled, and confusing, due to many reasons, our living becomes messy. Our ill-health, some chronic while some acute or random, daily living is messy as we feel stuck. I've lived through it and I knew it well but not more than you.

There are university students who messed up by joining the wrong course. The wrong course, I called it, because it's a promising subject but not interesting or tougher than expected. Yet there's no point of turning back as it involves both time and money. It can be depressing being stuck in one's own mess.

Many times in my life, I messed things up, especially when the trajectory of life takes the upper turn. In my imperfect life, I did things unnecessarily and necessarily messed with critical idealistic turns. Further, there are times when God seems unfair, messing around, but with a purpose only.

As you know now, we are messing with each other in our daily living. It has its positive side too. The positive side is when our messing with each other translates into concerns and connections. This messy living allows us to live in a society or neighborhood which created a welfare state.

The **negative side** becomes an obstacle in our living. We must take utmost care not mess the life of others. Our small words, careless whispers, and little careless act could destroy their good relationship; make someone's good day gone bad. So we can at least try not messing in an undesired way.

On a larger scale, we have this dogmatic practice of messing with each other as state and non-state actors. Our diplomatic outreach or campaigns between states are such examples. The hegemony of developed and economically stable countries in and around their neighboring states is another way of messing around. However, we are talking about the mess and messing on very petty issues yet large enough to mess up our entire living.

Here we will see kinds of mess in our messy life and beyond.

Evil Messing With Us:

Evil, in other words, the work of Satan, has been messing people's life since ages. The mode, methodology, and medium of operation might differ yet it troubled our living. As a kind of success test, the lives of many faithful people are also messed with.

Joseph's life had witnessed detours, trials, and temptations. His pilgrimage from his father's house to the pit; from the pit as a slave; to a successful man in the house of Potiphar, an officer of Pharaoh's, must be tough. However, Satan messed with him through Potiphar's wife, which downgraded and welcome a stint in prison. (Genesis 39)

David's household was a mess, in certain times, once he was messed by the work of evil in his personal life. Swords were drawn in the household, which saw him losing his beloved sons. It takes mournful of tears and time in untangling the mess. Yet David turned to the Lord, in his chaotic parts of life. (2 Sam. 22: 26-37)

Messing With God:

We might be witty, intelligent, and in a good position to handle issues but it's so wrong to mess with God. God's plans are always greater than the knowledge of mankind. However, in certain times we try messing, becoming the much-needed tool for the Evil's work.

Jonah, the small time prophet, had clear instruction from the Lord to do Him a favor. On his way, he messed it up which saw him going through difficult times, inside and outside the interior of the big fish.

But the Lord still fulfilled His mission saving the dwellers of Nineveh. It was sorry for Jonah to mess with God.

Simon, who is called Peter, was with his Teacher when he predicted His death on the cross and Resurrection. Sincere in his love for His teacher, Peter rebuked Jesus. "Never Lord, he said, "this shall never happen to you."

And he realized his messing with God's purpose when Jesus said to him, "Get behind me, Satan!" When we have mere concerns things of men or human, sometimes, we messed with God's plan.

Greater than the Mess:

It is true many people are buried in the deep waters of our messy living. We messed up our life very easily. Hardly do we possessed the wisdom to manage our careers and plans in this fast pace of life. It is quite understandable that we do not want to be left behind. And in this struggle we, many times, messed up our living.

Once we're messed things up, it is hard to untangle ourselves. And I write this because I too messed up living big time. The more we try, sometimes, the more tangled our living. It has an impact on our own life and our immediate family and friends. When all the laws of the land, traditions, and rituals cannot save us, Jesus Christ can save us.

Our problematic messy living, many times, messed the plans and purpose of God. At some point, it led us to rebuke and question God whether by destroying our relationship with Him or heighten our resentment of His work. However, we still can go to Him to save our messy living.

Our life might be messy, but God is greater than all the mess we created or we've been through. In Him, we are not consumed by our messy life once we turned to Him. Circumstances will remind us of the failures and difficulties we have had by messing with our thinking mind. Yet we can take refuge in Him.

Wrestle Living

Wrestling, like a game or sports, did not interest me much. For the sake of knowing the sport and in admiration of their hard work, I'd watched the game. It's a tiresome sporting adventure but when their hard work really paid off, it can change their fortune.

By definition, to wrestle is to force someone into a particular position by grappling with them. As a sport, it involves combat and grappling the opponent trying to cut-out their advances and manipulating their strength in forcing or throwing them on the ground. When some athletes can't throw the game because of injury, I empathized them.

In these games and sports, to simply put it, the player must try and brought down the opponent who is trying his best to refrain from falling down. Grappling and toppling the unwilling, in normal practices, is never easy. It takes lots of efforts and tactics to uproot a well-built person.

The recent release of the Bollywood (Hindi Film Industry) blockbuster, **Dangal** (Wrestling Competition) in India represents the hard work of wrestlers behind the scenes for us who did not access into their training podium. The hard works and inspirations, which would take them into the beautiful yet tension-filled wrestling bouts in the world of sports.

The movie, Dangal, follows the life of freestyle wrestlers, the Phogat family, from Balali Villages in Bhiwani District, Haryana, India. The Phogat Sisters, who were trained by their father, went on to win gold medals in different editions of Commonwealth Wrestling Championships.

This biographical drama film depicts the plight of a father who vows to realize his dream by training his daughters after he failed to secured gold medals for his country. In other words, it is about a family who tries to grapple their fortune despite the struggles it takes.

In the game of life, in some way, we are presented in the wrestling bout as our everyday life is filled with struggles. Some struggled with lifelong depression, poverty, wrestled with the inner voice, ill-health, and many more. We are Challengers of the world so that we'd not get defeated in this bout of life.

It might seem disheartening to present it this way. And I know that sometimes it's too much of our struggles, for weak persons like me, competing in this game of life. However, that's the reality of life. And it's really difficult to meet the requirements of this life should we wanted to live on.

Wrestling Living:

Since the day of our inception, we wrestle for our survival. The babies born in an unsterile place started wrestling for pumping air into the lungs which would ignite life. In this crucial period, failure to pumped-in air by way of idling would prove detrimental for a new life.

The zeal for living, the zeal to go on, provides the heart of a wrestler in our daily life. Should we remain idle, accepting failures in the midst of time, we'd surely lost the game. I cannot say with certainty that all our acts and struggles would pay off which would turn us into successful persons, but without struggling our bits we'd get into deeper mud of life. So, it is necessary at least for our survival.

In almost every game, timing and techniques decide the winner. As we put it earlier, there are things in life which mess with us, which needs to be toppled or thwarted in the most appropriate time. And without doing so, the reverse advantage will consume our life. Grappling and toppling Satan without the help of God wouldn't be easy.

The Man Who Wrestle With God:

After his staying days with Laban were over, Jacob headed back to his land to meet his brother Esau. He sent his servants to meet Esau before him, as he's still unsure whether his brother would accept him. So he stayed alone in his camp nearby Jabbok throughout the night.

There, in the darkness of the night, a man (an angel as recorded in Hosea 12:4) wrestled with him till daybreak. When the man saw he could not overpower him, he touched the socket of Jacob's hip pleading to let him go. But Jacob replied, "I will not let you go unless you blessed me." (Genesis 32:22-31)

It was a game-changer moment for him as the man blessed him there. The man changes his name from Jacob to Israel, because Jacob struggled with God and with humans and overcame him. This man wrestled with anything that comes in his way turning his obstacles into a source of blessings.

Jacob's wrestle with God was a struggle, in his loneliness, which makes his life worthy. He was still unsure whether his bother would accept him or not. If not, what would be his next step, he must have been in a dilemma and insecure.

What Do You Wrestle With?

Before we were born, we're not even asked, the game is set. And the technique of winning the game is also given. Many before us and even after us will win the game. What do we wrestle with today depends on our mindset? Do we wrestle for more of our personal gain or for the love of God?

Today, it would be a joyous moment if we wrestle with God as it would draw us closer to Him. It would make us wanting more of Him. We know that we can't topple or mess with God's plan but by begging and holding firmly on God and His promises, God would give us the desires of our heart.

The Bible says, "Our struggle is not against flesh and blood, but against the rulers, against the powers, against the world forces of this darkness, against the spiritual forces of wickedness in the heavenly places." (Ephesians 6:12) Wow! That'll be hard, someone quips. And it is true. However, with the help of the Spirit, we'll win the struggle.

It is worth living as there are instances and elements to wrestle with. These wrestling bouts make us know more of the might of God. **"It is finished!"** declared Jesus Christ on the cross. (John 19:30) And the time will soon come when we enjoy victorious life in its entirety.

Wrestling with life and its consequences by following the instruction given in the manual book - the Holy Bible, is the only way in winning the bout, righting the wrongs. May the grace and mercy of God be with us to everyone wrestling the work of evil!

Let us not simply throw the game without fighting. We better squeeze our strength fighting the opponents as our Abiding Savior did. We would indeed prevail in the right time and in the right place.

Chapter Eleven

In His biding Grace: The Joy of Living

I am obligated to talk about the abiding grace showered upon me. Synonyms of abiding are: enduring, persisting, long-lasting, lifelong, unending, constant, stable, unchanging, and many more. While grace in its verb form is also used as dignify, bestow honor, favor, enhance, and the likes.

Here in this series, I wanted to emphasize 'His abiding grace'. God's grace and favor are enduring as well as unending. We are bestowed with many good things, some are considered small, and taken for granted.

The Joy of Breathing

The Joy of Breathing has been revealed in my journey of life. Breath-holding games - who can hold longer by diving in water or in the open air, are popular in my childhood. However, we did not think so much about breathing because it seems so normal.

Read this: I was unconscious. I can't feel the oxygen mask being attached to my nose. It was supposed to increase my oxygen intake, in case I didn't get enough. Frankly speaking, the doctors know my condition is critical and they are doing whatever they could!

Taking you back a few hours; it was a fine winter morning. We were strolling and getting fresh air in the park nearby. Getting home, I

73

decided to take rest. I could sense something is wrong in my body. Something unusual is taking place.

I wanted to take as much air as I can, and I know, I need more air. However, the more I tried to breathe in the more difficult it was. Air did not want to enter through my nostril nor my mouth! It was more than tiresome.

The feeling was hard to put in words. In short, I remained unconscious in a few minutes. Several hours of battling for life ensued. However, in the end, my God spared, what I called, my life. I'm alive! In the past, I couldn't recall myself thanking God for the air I'd breathed in.

The oxygen, the entire volume of oxygen, intake for my living was *free of cost!* I must be thankful! I was filled with great joy, indeed. I did not ask for these things: to provide fresh air, to regulate my breathing process, in particular.

Now, I realized I was getting beyond what I could ask for. It gives me immense pleasure and joy, to breathe take in the air freely. When in need, it was costly to buy oxygen. We must be joyful for what we get!

In today's world, we feel blessed and happy only when we acquired big things that are expensive. We value based on the cost of them. Very small things, it seems, but think of them and be happy. So, breathe in as much air as you can or while you can.

The Joy of Sleeping

It was well past midnight. I close my eyes but I did not sleep. I am in my thirties, not old as yet. My normal body functioning has changed, some years ago.

Just one mistake, I did not take my medicine in time. My body needs rest. My mind needs rest. And the pain will ease. If I didn't get enough sleep, a more serious problem might follow.

I was, already, warned about the possible consequences during my hospital stay, and I knew that too. When we were young and healthy, sleepiness comes too soon - even before we were ready! I wanted to read more but felt too sleepy to go on.

Before I knew it, it was morning! When morning comes, I woke up fresh - hale, and hearty because of the good night's sleep – rested well. Get ready for the day's work humming music with a huge smile.

Yet, when I thank God for the good night sleep, I tend to rush through it. I hardly pause for a moment to let my heart be filled with joy from up above. The happiness was priceless.

God's abiding grace, which was bestowed upon me, I hardly gave sincere thought. The night in my bed, turning from side-to-side, I'd **battled** for sleep and rest. It was not as easy as it seems. It was a gift from God.

When I can't sleep in time, the night seems to be a long dark period of life. One night feels like a year of drought where everyone is deprived of good harvest, which would eventually lead to unrest. But still, in those sleepless nights, when I can sense the Lord's presence; my heart rested.

However, the body witnessed strain eyes and sleep-deprived body ache. The Lord gives sleep to His beloved. Sleep gives us rest! Medicine-induced sleep is tiresome and non-enjoyable. Several times I'd experienced it.

More than that, sedation is hard to bear when you wake up. I have been through it, and I could say, I knew it. The one gifted by God is all special more than we know.

To sleep and be able to wake up again is the greatest gift of all. It signifies the superiority of the living God. The day will come when we won't wake up again. I lay down and when I woke up the Lord is still with me. When I won't wake up again, that day, I'll be with my Savior!

Once again, sleep is a wonderful gift we get from God. And to wake up again is even more beautiful. It is because of His abiding or enduring grace, which cannot be bought. God's abiding grace is sufficient for all, especially to His children in Christ. His grace is priceless!

The Joy of Sharing in Suffering

When we suffered hardships in life, we wanted someone to talk to. And, that too, if we're able to talk. We wanted to pour out our sufferings by letting it out.

There is no joy to any types of suffering yet there can be a joy to any types of suffering. Personally, I'd been through some hardships and suffering and from the people I met on the way. Let's discuss some of them.

Not all people understand our inner feeling. Most people tend to hide within us. People are afraid to share their sufferings with any random person. We need someone trustworthy, understanding, and not repulsive in nature. Yet it is hard to find.

There are some who could simply react to your sufferings in one sentence - blunt and plain. For, they do not know what is burning inside someone's life. However, it would be wise not to react or question someone suffering any pain, be it emotional, physical, or even in grief.

When we are in the suffering mode, our mind roamed around leading us to happiness and sadness, inside our heart. This resulted in changes in mood frequently, which sometimes becomes unbearable for us and our surroundings.

It is a privilege, I could say, to meet several people I have known in their sufferings and talked with them. Some get comforted and find joy in their suffering as it will not last forever. There will be an end to sufferings although in different ways.

Years ago, my father was diagnosed with cancer. It left us in great distress. We do not know what is before us yet we expect something worst to happen as the suffering is life-threatening. That same year, we learned that I would be undergoing brain surgery due to my prolonged neurological disorder.

My father was done with his first round of Chemotherapy when I was operated upon. Unfortunately yet maybe God willing, my father and I become a suffering partner to whom we can deeply let out our sufferings. We talked about so many things. Let me lay out some of them here:

About The End:

Death has been the subject of our sharing, sometimes. We reassured each other of what lies ahead. Being both of us enjoying the Salvation of Jesus Christ, we are determined to meet Him in the near future.

In the course of time, I'd brushed with death, which I gladly share with my father and my families. There is a far better place waiting for us to enjoy. No science and technology needed to proof or help but the blood of Christ, shed many many years ago, was sufficient to get us there.

I remember my father calling me over the phone one particular day. He told me, "I thought my end has been approaching. The time has come to be with Him. I can sense death calling. But I am not afraid to go. However, it is not time yet!" I could sense him smiling while telling me this. He was laughing although tired, during our conversation. It was a great relief to hear that! And we rejoice in praising the Lord for such comfort. A year ago, his time has finally come. My dear father, see you in Heaven!

About Life:

We did talk about life a lot, in some way as a special child of God. There are several things we wanted to re-do or make-over but that's not possible. So far, the sufferings we had are for our own life; very less for others around us. Yet if God blessed upon our sufferings, it can be useful. And we prayed for that too.

'The special child of God,' we called ourselves. Yes, there is nothing special about not being able to lead a normal life, at least for a while. I will tell you why we called ourselves a special child of God.

In our suffering, we talked to God more often. We need Him every minute and every hour to be with us. Whatever happens and whatever comes our way, if God is with us, the rest we worry not. We wanted to be in touch with Him all the time.

More so, our heart becomes more open to Him ever than before. His words are more penetrating than usual. We are in fellowship with our Savior. He looked after every minute details of our lives and He is always close by – within reach. To the suffering soul, He is always near.

Does God Really Care?

Jesus Christ's prayer for His disciples and all believers in John 17:6-25, I remembered, we discussed in a lengthy conversation. We also get comforted by His prayer – the Prayer of the Lord to His Father. He is still praying for us in the same way or even more than before.

In this prayer, it is clear that Jesus Christ knew exactly what we are going through. He Himself lived in this world in our human form. The pain, sufferings, hardships, He knew it all. He'd been through it. He'd seen it all. And now that's very comforting.

Although I wanted to discuss these verses in great detail, let me pick some in between here. These are the prayer Jesus Christ had for us. Please go through them: *"While I was with them, I protected them and kept them safe by that name you gave me."* (Verse 12a) He really did. He saved them from their physical sickness and even from death.

"My prayer is not that you take them out of the world but that you protect them from the evil one. They are not of the world, even as I am not of it." (Verses 15 and 16) Our sufferings are allowed but not to cause us to harm beyond we can stand.

The One who doesn't belong to this world had gone through sufferings. So, we must also endure some sufferings. But He will protect us from the evil one.

"I have made you known to them, and will continue to make you known in order that the love you have for me may be in them and that I myself may be in them." (Verse 26) This is exactly what He did. Made known to us and He will never let us suffer alone being Him within us.

We get comforted with these verses in the midst of our sufferings. When we would find the implications and express it out there can be joyous moments.

Becoming a Partner in Sufferings:

Everyone needs someone to talk to, to let out to someone trustworthy while in sufferings. For me, most unexpected, unfortunate or uncalled for, my father becomes my suffering partner. Being both of us suffering we can almost fully understand each other.

Sometimes full of hope, the other time with less hope - the mind of a suffering person can be unsteady. Anyone can fit in as a partner, someone who will listen to them. One does not need prior training. We have God-given quality to do so if we are willing. You can be one of them.

For those sufferers who do not have someone to share their mind, Our God is there to listen. Not only listen, But He also acts upon our cases too. Although His ways are beyond what men can understand. Not acting or doing something the way we desired does not mean that God is not working. He is always at work.

Lastly, I did not finish my race yet, but I write because I hope it might be useful.

To Timothy, Apostle Paul wrote, "I have fought the good fight, I have finished the race, I have kept the faith." (2 Timothy 4:7) This was written shortly before Paul's death.

Although, Apostle Paul's sufferings were way beyond my sufferings, which I firmly believe. When I finished this world of suffering, I wanted to say the same with my head held high.

The Joy of Companionship

In moments of sadness and happiness, we always need someone's company to be with us.

'Companion' in its verb form could be 'accompany' with whom one spends lots of time with or travel with. Synonyms of 'companionship' are friendship, acquaintance, togetherness, and many more.

We do know that God is always with us. His abiding grace is sufficient. But many times, we cannot feel His companion right away. To feel it, first, we need to empty ourselves and give Him, His much deserved, space. Surely, He will make us whole again.

Let me share you part of my journal entry: June 14, 2017, 1400 hours. As usual, some unwanted occurrence visited me. This time, it's a bit harder. But I try to let it pass as soon as possible. It might be due to the change in weather condition, I guess, as it happened before.

We were at home with my two little children. I let them know of my situation and that God's abiding grace will be with us.

I kneel down to pray to slide on our bed. My eyes got a bit blurry but I was fine. My little ones did not want to disturb me.

They came, and as we pray, I hold them in my arms – one on my left and the other on my right. I told them to put their holy hands on my head and pray for me too. And they did!

"Heal my daddy's head inside-out. Please give daddy longevity. So that we will live together for a long time. We love him very much!"

On hearing their prayer, it gives me new strength and I was filled with tears of happiness. It gives me the strength to carry on.

Then I resume my prayer and thank God for everything. His companionship came in the form of my own children today! I am really hopeful that my God would consider their request.

We cannot, always, have the same strength as yesterdays. It might be due to different reasons. Small things, for some other persons, can still let us down. As long as we are breathing, it will exist.

When we were discouraged and disturbed, we want a companion, at least. But, if you're like me, we don't want to let loose our mind and everything either.

Today, in what form do you get your companion – that, I did not know. However, our heavenly father is and was so kind to be with us. It is just that we don't have time to realize His presence.

It reminded me of how Elisha was prompted to ask God to open the eyes of his servant to see 'the invisible'! (2 Kings 6: 14-17)

In moments of loneliness and helplessness, several times, we wanted to see 'the Invisibles', if you're like me. For a person who easily gets disturbed because of the long-suffering and not living the dream, we wanted to feel His presence, His abiding companionship, every day and every hour.

For the wandering mind, the companionship of someone is most needed. For the insecure at heart, it gives relief with someone's mere companion. This is one among the JOY of living in abiding grace.

Do not fear. He will keep you safe and sound, in His companionship.

The Joy of Experiencing Hallucination

In my journey of life, several times, I'd experienced hallucinations due to health-related problems.

Those series are not my cherished moments yet it is worth recalling in counting God's abiding grace. In some ways, it is beneficial to me, in the walk of life.

Hallucination may mean, a state of mind or experience involving apparent perception which is not real. Synonyms of hallucination are an illusion, delusion, mirage, delirium, and many more.

Let me share you just one instance of the experience:

We were dealing with finance and accounting jobs in the office during those days. In the middle of the day, we can be very busy with our work usurping our mind and energy. The stage was set for my hallucination, and I never knew that.

Being in the capital city of India, Hindi and English is the spoken language, although Hindi edge over English here. At an instance, it suddenly seems that all the persons near me are speaking in one tongue. That too, my native tongue and the likes, which was spoken in my hometown some thousand miles away!

This time my vision was not blurred, as I feel it. It's just that the language is spoken or what I heard that makes the difference. Hallucinating, in some ways, the experiences one had gone through can be dissimilar.

The situation was uncontrollable and I seemed to enjoy the atmosphere, as I did not know that I was hallucinating. It was beyond what one could do something.

Still, I was busy working on my computer when it stops happening. Workplace colleagues helped me get home that day.

Several wrong financial transactions were made by me in that short span of time. But then, God's abiding grace is sufficient for me as there was no such transaction, which cannot be rectified. The occurrence helped me realized the so many good sides of my colleagues.

These few problems showed more of the goodness of my friends. Many times, they sent me home or helped me out.

More importantly, it is a huge privilege to be able to wake up from hallucinating. There is very less or almost nothing one could do when it really happens. It is because of God's abiding grace only, that we could be living. That's one among the joys of living.

It gives me the joy to be alive and tell the tales of my mild sufferings till now. Yet I am more thankful for everything that we have experienced.

But one thing, in our semi-conscious state, sometimes we tend to utter things which are less valuable. So, dear readers, enjoy the joy of living life to its fullest extent while you can.

And, always remember, you might be more blessed, than some of us, to not have gone through sufferings which might hamper your being. Be happy and stay blessed.

His grace is abiding and/or enduring, God knows what is best for us! Yet it is difficult to say that all the time. Altogether, it constituted, what is called, the Joy of Living!

The Joy of Getting Closer

In my younger days, I loved to read as much as I could. I'd enjoyed being submerged in thoughts of wise people. In my innate being, I wanted to know more about them, personally.

Let me confessed a little bit, I'd follow a few communists whose writing pattern had become an obsession to me. I'd imitate their styles during my school days. More than the content in their writing, it is their style of expressing, I had enjoyed.

We all enjoyed learning new things, I hope, for which writers or columnist became our channel for getting useful information and resources.

Few years had passed, when I got to know more about their ideologies and personal ethics, I stopped following some of them. I am no more a huge fan of them. Why? Because, only in my perception, I know them enough to the extent to even dislike them.

That being said, there are a few reasons – I have become more critical of them. And I remained there, to be among their faultfinders before I've moved on.

Now, getting to know more and getting closed are quite similar yet dissimilar hugely. And as you see, getting to know more of someone does not end in being getting close, somehow or never.

In the affairs of our so-called 'love life or romance', we can be attracted to someone before knowing them as much as we wanted to. It can lead to a spark between two different people meeting in the stages of life - infatuation.

There are some who are unable to tolerate and enjoyed their incompatibility, which gradually let them split despite their past commitments to each other. Failed partnership, a failed marriage, failed relationship, or whatever name we called them.

In reality, our getting to know more must have led us to be getting closer. However, it can hit rock bottom and blow wide open otherwise. There's nothing as such 'an incompatibility-proof' in all matters.

What is next? Being unable to get closer because of the 'I know you' attitude, jealousy plays a spoiler. When we felt not close enough for a few moments, our innate evil owner could creep in, destroying everything we had.

This critical view of fault finding can turn into compassion! One can take joy in dealing with incompatibility. When compassion creeps in, criticisms can turn us into being closer.

One thing, I must tell you, in the love of God poured out and made available in the blood of Jesus Christ, all things are made possible in His might.

Remember all the divisive barriers and personal strongholds were crashed on the Cross of Calvary, in His abiding grace.

Apostle Paul urged the believers, of Philippians, to let their knowledge and insights must draw them closer to the resurrected Christ. When he wrote to them, in Philippians 1:9, "And this is my prayer that your love may abound more and more in knowledge and depth of insight."

Our God, always, remained close in His abiding grace. The more we know the more we get closer or want to get closer instead.

Unlike other personalities and existing creatures of God, we could be as close as Christ Jesus, and as much as we wanted to. His arm is always open to anyone. Let me end herewith;

To know more of Christ is to become closer to Him, day by day!

The Joy of Having Visitors

Sometimes, our relatives visited us. In the city where we now lived, we have few relatives. When they can spare some time to visit us we were really happy and excited.

The children are busy playing their games together. It was a good feeling for them to get to know each other. For the parents, it was a good time to share about life as we faced it, which could provide us with valuable lessons to take care for the future.

We are happy because we have someone who loves spending time with us. The conversations could be endless as we jumped from one topic to another. Moreover, when we have the chance to meet old friends and old neighbors, we have so many things to let out.

Time for Visitation:

Time for visitations cannot be bought. We cannot coerce someone to visit us either. It is a priceless experience. To the visitors during my hospital stay, I am more than grateful. Yet due to my health conditions, I am unable to talk to them at that time.

In our hard times, God had sent his people, in His abiding grace, to help us in prayers even inside the hospital. When in grief, the presence of visitors and relatives make the suffering a bit easier. The face of God, for comfort, can be seen in the face of our visitors and the warmth can be felt too.

Further, let me broadly classify visitors into two: the uninvited visitors and the invited visitors.

The Uninvited Visitors:

The other name for uninvited visitors could be 'the crashers' in weddings and personal events. First, let's talk about *'Gatecrashers'*. A Gate Crasher is a person who attends some event or social affair without being invited or without having proper credentials to get in. Some do it to gain popularity while some gate crashed to disrupt the atmosphere of an event or party.

Second, *Wedding Crashers* must be the one who is most unwelcome. Wedding Crashers can be chaotic and unpredictable. If you have already watched the Hollywood movie 'Wedding Crashers' and its sequel, you already knew it.

Third, having visitors like the 'Dupree' of the Hollywood movie 'You, me and Dupree' can be annoying at times. However, it can be useful in some way or the other. Our toleration level might get boosted.

Above all, visitors unannounced can create nuisance although the intention and purpose might be good. And the unwanted situation could be saved by letting our visits known beforehand.

The Invited Visitors:

"My Lord, if I have found favor in Your sight, do not pass on by Your servant," Abraham pleaded the three men standing by the terebinth tree of Mamre. They obliged and, in short, he fed them. The three men promised to return in time. They were on their way to Sodom and Gomorrah.

They told Abraham, that, "Sarah your wife shall have a son." After which, the three men rose from there and looked towards Sodom.

(Genesis 18) Thus, the due promise of Abraham becoming a mighty nation came true. Since he had invited the three visitors in his tent, he was blessed. To be noted here; Abraham invited them.

Two, two men were walking on the Road to Emmaus. They were lonely and sad; they believed that the Messiah would redeem Israel here on earth. But Jesus Christ was crucified before their very eyes. Then, a stranger joined them.

They invited Him saying, "Abide with us, for it is toward evening, the day is far spent." And He went in to stay with them. He sat with them at the table. He blessed and broke the bread before their very eyes. And behold, it was their master, Jesus Christ who had been resurrected from the death. (Luke 24:13-31)

Now, consider this: should we let ourselves to be left annoyed by the uninvited visitors or invited a visitor before it is late?

In this lonely world, should we invite Jesus Christ; He is ready to abide with us. He would warmth our heart, filled our emptiness and makes us whole again.

Christ has unlimited time for visitations yet we have to take a decision and invite Him. Since our eyes are opened – knowing good and evil - after what had happened in the Garden of Eden. In other words, since the time we have been deceived.

On our part, it is our duty to invite Him; not to let him pass on by and feed us from His own hand. Thereafter, He would get us filled and work in us, according to our needs.

The Joy of Letting Go

Our thought process, sometimes, is beyond our control. Our innate being has been blessed with great diversity, which altogether made up a sane being. God's abiding grace makes the necessary adjustments in our life.

Memories formed an important part of our living. Memories help us retain good and bad things we came across. We cannot simply let go of anything on our own nor can we retain memories on our own. It seems so normal but it is not. Another word for letting it go might be forgiven.

Forgiveness comes from the Lord. When we can forgive and forget, we find inner peace. We can achieve it by being in the Lord. The power of forgiveness works wonders in every life.

Forgetfulness, or being forgetful, is another thing which might hamper our living. But in its normal tempo, we find rest and get a good night sleep. Imagine your thinking process did not stop before going to sleep, it would be, and is, very tiresome. In this context, we must be thankful to God for being forgetful.

As a normal human being, I hope, we have certain occurrences which we don't want to let go. It might be hurtful to us yet we don't want to let go either. Since all our ventures or adventures in the journey of life cannot yield good results, this kind of things happened. Even after we have learned lessons from previous mistakes, it can still come to haunt us. However, by being covered up in His abiding grace, we can lessen the aftereffects.

Letting it go helps us living past our dark period of life. It is true that one can never preplan our journey of life in its minute details. Sometimes the 'very much' unexpected person or occurrence, outside of our normal life, can still hurt us at the least expected time and place. Still, this is life and we should be able to filter it and try letting it go.

In our completely broken state, most of life's lessons are best learned. Let me interrupt you here: I am not saying that I'm a learned person. Should you be saying, you're living in your perfect world, I must agree with you too. It is because you possess that power of letting it go under His abiding grace.

Ostensibly, the hardest part of life is letting it go of the memories of loved ones who are gone way too soon. Although they are gone, we tend to cherish them in our minds. It is a good thing to remember them, yet it might lead to bitterness in living. Take it all to the Lord; all will be fine in His abiding grace. However, it should be noted that no human mind could fully understand the Lord's way.

Should someone hurt you try letting go without hurting them back. Hurting back benefits none. And it simply let our lives miserable. By not hurting back, we seem to be a loser, but in reality, it benefitted us. It is more closure to Christ-likeness also. It gives us insurmountable pain, to not let go of something, which was already gone.

It also applies to something that wanted to go, yet we still want to keep it. If it is difficult, ask God for help. It is the most difficult part of life, especially, if it happens before we get ready. There is power in letting go of certain bitter memories. It can give us tremendous joy - the joy of living or the joy of letting it go.

Let me end herewith the greatest joy of letting it go: Jesus Christ paid the price for our sins. To one who is willing to accept that He forgives and forget his sins. He took away our past sinful life. We became a new creation in Him. He let go of our, any amount of, previous transgressions!

This is the greatest Joy of Living we are bestowed through God's abiding grace!

The Joy of Finding the Zeal for Living

It is my prerogative in His abiding grace; to always start my days with, at least one verse from, the Scripture. It renewed my hope, giving me the zeal of living, even in my worst circumstances. There are times though when I go by my own conveniences getting absorbed in other things.

At times, my minds got usurped by what is happening around us. Too much focusing on the happening around us might distort our zeal of living. Some of the Synonyms of zeal are passion, enthusiasm, eagerness, fervor, love, and many more. In brief, zeal can be defined as the energy or enthusiasm in pursuit of a cause.

In my free time, I would glance around the world through printed media. Hate-crimes are rampant in every corner of the world. The flamboyant lifestyles of some people adversely affect thousands of people, either directly or indirectly. Distortion of facts, even in religious matter, to suit one's living and in fulfilling their selfish ambitions becomes a threat to humankind.

More and more people claimed to follow God by only befitting or letting down their faith. Spreading false prophecy, distorting anything on the way; by way of playing the so-called diplomacy has been disheartening. Each day we are closer to the end of time. Especially to those who do not have a hope of "life after death" or unmoved by the promise of life after death, they are in their prime.

In a world of distorted conscience, if I do not believe in the promised privilege about our eternal glory after death, it would be disturbing to spend each day. What really does the world has to offer? It is for you to think.

It might sound unwise to someone who enjoyed fitting in the systems of the world, as it is. I have been through some of the enjoyment but it's not worth it. In the end, you wanted more. Either you ended up with guilty feeling or you get stuck. Our body has been in its declining mode once it reached its peak.

However, our mental strength in keeping our faith just started heading towards maturity. Jesus Christ, the Son of God, states, "I am the resurrection and the life. He who believes in Me, though he may die, he shall live" (John 11:25)

The time, for my Savior to take me home, is worth waiting. Getting home - from a journey full of challenges and unfulfilled dreams – that's the reason behind getting the zeal to live on. For someone who is really in Him, life is not a burden but enjoyment. Should you ask me how do I still have hope and have the zeal to go on?

By now, I hope, you get it right. Faith, without His abiding grace, would get lost on the way. Yet even when there seems my faith has been lost, in His grace it gets renewed again and again. Consider the word of the resurrected Christ in these verses, even before His Crucifixion: "Because I live, you will live also" (John 14:19).

Jesus Christ had also taught His disciples, His intention, for all of mankind: "I have come that they may have life and that they may have it more abundantly" (John 10:10)

So that our lives may not be consumed by sufferings, but have a great zeal of leaning towards him.

The Joy of Finding Hope Amidst Uncertainty

Uncertainty, undeniably, is one of the ingredients in the walk of life. It happened for a reason, maybe.

One day, my son just came back from school. As usual, I enquired as to what they did at school. They played and they enjoyed, which was good. When we sent our children to school, we want them to learn something.

If their progress can be seen, we become happier. Anyways, it doesn't happen that way, always. Some worksheets, they brought along, needs to be done at home. At times, children simply didn't follow our instructions. And we forget they are just starting. As a parent, we are uncertain about their future.

Parenting was never easy - you get discouraged one minute, you get happy with full of hope the other time. Imparting knowledge, for some of us, isn't easy. That's why we sent them to school, to get help while we raised them.

We want our children to blossom into stars. However, several rounds of 'test of patience' needed to overcome first. Amidst that uncertainty, we have hope when we rested the matter in God's Abiding Grace.

Uncertainty in Investments:

Investments, in all its forms, had an uncertain future. The salesperson tries to feed us a good return for every policy or investment plans. It is their job; they are trained for that purpose only. It is us, the investors, who got stuck if it goes awry.

We might not reap the fruit in time. Like others, in our pursuit of happiness, we tend to invest amidst uncertainty. We must take a risk yet it can take us into bondage. Being unable to get rid of any investments due to unforeseen reasons is also hard to bear.

Yet, in His abiding grace, we have hope that at least we might be delivered in time. In any type of outcome, God's grace is behind what led us today.

Emptiness, inside the heart, can eat up our body too. Several times, when I wanted to commune with God, it seems God was far away today. When our emptiness is not filled by the Holy Spirit, it is as good as a half-dead person. When the cup is not filled, we have nothing to offer our surroundings.

In this time of uncertainty, God's abiding grace still abided with us although we did not feel it. We wanted to perform good things yet we ended up doing bad things. Without His grace, not a soul will live. Waiting silently to transform us, to fill us again, will give us hope amidst this uncertainty – the dilemma or unpredictability.

Uncertainty in phases of life:

When we're let down or we felt let down beyond our normal living, it is more difficult. One evening, as usual, we go out to spend time in a park nearby. My children, in their prime, were active. They wanted to play with me. At times, I am unable to play with them as much as they wanted. It isn't easy to be in that condition.

For every person, I hope, it is our dream to spent time with, play with our children till they get bored. It was uncertain when would Daddy get fully fit to play with them into their heart's contentment.

Yet you don't want to let them know of all your difficulties. It's their happiness that comes first.

Time and again, it is my duty to give them hope and assured them of His abiding grace. One thing is certain amidst all uncertainty, Jesus Christ died for us. He set the path right for all of us.

Let me end herewith that in every sphere of uncertainty in our walk of life, God's grace is abiding. He did all the necessities unseen to our earthly eyes. It's just that we didn't observe God's work or might be ignoring it. Let's try to make uncertainty be just a phase in our journey.

Chapter Twelve

Many Questions; Few Answers

It's no surprise when my children have many questions to ask; even to the answers, I did not know. I wanted to give them legitimate answers because they remember everything all well. One thing is certain; there are big things to make it so easy and small without losing their taste.

On my part, it is important to maintain vivacity of the subject, as they get distracted easily. However, they'd come back with the same question a few other time. And this time for sure, they needed an answer. By the way, I'm spending my time with them 24/7.

In the morning, just before they set out from school, our prayer time was perturbed by my nauseous feel or vomiting. When they enquired, I do have an answer to explain the problem; it's the side effects of the medicine I've taken for more than a decade.

However, what I cannot tell my children is the time I will get over this problem. These are the things we must leave it to our God, I'd tell them when my son readily prayed for my well being first thing first in the morning.

Well, there are some questions I can readily answer. For example, the question relating to my childhood days, except the name of a few friends. What would happen if we take fish out of the water, and why? What would be my birthday gift this year? And so on.

Coming to a little bit tougher questions: why do leaves turn into yellow before they fall down? For a child who's not been into

101

Photosynthesis as yet, it takes time to explain. When he's satisfied with my answer, we leave it at that; satisfaction is the key.

A few months ago, my son developed a keen interest in the planetary system. We even wanted to go there and examined them if the existing theories and hypothesis, which I have read, were right should there be oxygen in outer space. Please take it slow; it's from children's point of view.

The directions of the blowing wind, he asked me. With the help of the weatherman, I can answer that question. Yet long before the live update of the weatherman, King Solomon of Israel already knew it because God has given him wisdom.

We took turns showing the satellite pictures, from ISS, till we get satisfied. It's just wonderful how they spin and revolt around the sun, we noted. But greater than the system was the Creator, the Creator of everything discovered and not yet discovered by humanity.

These are a few glimpses of my time with my children as well as what I wanted to convey here. Standing on the bright side of life, many answers he will found in his quest for the wisdom of a lifetime. However, it's a joy for me tickling or joyfully mocking their developing brain.

Few More Questions: Sovereignty of God

We wanted to know the reason for almost everything even if it doesn't benefit us. It is good, in one way, it means we wanted to gain knowledge.

How the earth did come into being? It is because God created it with a purpose. What would be the purpose? It is a place for us to enjoy the communion of God but we destroyed it. And we'll continue to destroy till the end.

How does God create everything? He created with His words; He said, "Let there be ….", in the first place. (Genesis 1) And in the same way, he created all things. There is no one who can create anything with words.

In a way that he'd be able to understand we discussed the resurrection of the dead. The resurrection of the dead and the separation of soul and body is governed by the supremacy of God. All powers are in the hands of the Lord.

In its simplest term, what we do not know reveals the Sovereignty of God behind our existence. Our God revealed his secret to the humble heart in their pilgrimage, preparing them for a time together with him in eternity.

The Sovereignty of God in Our Life:

In my journey filled with blessings, sufferings, and pain, sometimes, I felt blinded to see the plan and purpose of God for a useless person like me. It is I who had many questions yet some questions are better left unanswered.

We do not have records of a neurological disorder in the family, from both sides of the family, yet I still struggled with epilepsy. Although I'm almost getting over with it now, since it's been more than a decade long battle, I did ask my doctor the clear reason behind the illness.

Well, I admit that I have sinned against the Lord; but if it's supposed to be a punishment for my sins I won't live to write this anymore. My pain and sufferings are more of a blessing in a way that I spend more time relying on His words, in the Sovereignty of God, seen in His words.

Should I know all the reasons for every happening in and around me, I'd be on the same level with God which would mean I wouldn't need God. Thus my life is not good without God. There are things to be understood in later life.

Jacob, the biblical Jacob, asked several questions to Laban wondering the way he had treated him. Jacob has worked tirelessly for Laban, the father of his wives, yet he was mistreated. However, he knows that the Sovereign Lord ruled over his problems. God has a purpose; He was preparing him for good use of the blessing he had received.

Joseph's life story was no different. The revelations through his dreams were huge before he began his journey down from the pit to servanthood, servant to being humiliated for no sin of his until God raised him up.

God's sovereign plan was seen in the life of Joseph. He waited patiently trusting on the Lord.

The Sovereignty of God:

As it is necessary for me to respect the state and it's functionaries to maintain their sovereignty as I have been taught in my Political Science classes. More than that, I cannot and will not challenge the sovereignty of God if I accept to abide by the laws and regulations of my nation and the place where I am in.

Let God be what He is, for I know through his work and need no scientific research to prove his existence and Power. Instead, I will take comfort in His salvation.

I want God to surprise me with his secret supremacy in my arduous task of life. It is good to abide in the sovereign authority of God and we will praise him for that.

But now, there are many things I did not understand, for what I loss and grief, but I have a God who understands all. And the Lord gave me comfort although all my queries are not answered. In all his glory, it will be revealed soon.

The Answer; Sovereign Plan:

In the uncertainties of life more or his certainties he'd let me see. For, he wants a heart wholly dependent on him. And He is able to hold onto the heart's desire of man.

The Apostle Paul's imprisonment was a sovereign plan; his outburst says it all in Romans 11:33-36:

Oh, the depth of the riches of the wisdom and knowledge of God! How unsearchable his judgments, and his paths beyond tracing out! "Who has known the mind of the Lord? Or who has been his counselor?"
"Who has ever given to God, that God should repay them?" For from him and through him and for him are all things. To him be the glory forever! Amen.

For since the creation of the world God's invisible qualities—his eternal power and divine nature—have been clearly seen, being understood from what has been made, so that people are without excuse.

When we get few, or no answers at all, let us not lose heart. Lord, steer our life in the way of Yours. We want to know more about you!

Unchanging Amount of Love

"I am sorry. But this doesn't change the amount of love in the house," I said to my children while letting them do their homework, ending their free time for a moment.

There are times when I need to reiterate my love for them. I do love them, but when something goes wrong I need to intervene and take action. My interventions cannot, always, be sweet and welcomed by them.

Some **restrictions and limitations** need to be followed by me, which in my hope would extract the best out of them while preserving their innate quality. It is my obligation, as a parent, to guide them to the best of my knowledge and belief. (Proverbs 3:12)

We have this notion that the amount of love in the family gets depleted in due course of time. Time doesn't change the amount of love. We might not say *'I love you'* as much before as we did today. However, with each time passing by our love grew. And it's better to tell each other our love than not.

By not agreeing to every decision of ours, the amount of love doesn't change at all. They are sacrifices made for combating the unity of the family. Every member of the family contributes in different ways. If we could build a good family, it'd get reflected in society.

As we go on with our lives, there could be several factors which could make us think that the amount of love gets change. We met a different kind of people in our daily life who could influence, in good or bad, our way of thinking.

For example, **parenting** is a vast subject whose practicality depends massively on every father or mother. Our way of raising children might differ with our vision. Children are quick to spot the difference and for them, the grass always looks greener on the other side. We've been through it so it doesn't require detailed explanation.

It was not a good feeling being unable to play with my children, inside and outside the house. Leave aside playing, there are times when it is difficult speaking and talking with them due to some unwanted side effects of medicine intake. However, our amount of love doesn't change at all. It's just that our activities are limited.

What Amount of Love?

As we grow up, our parents have entrusted us to carry on with the instruction they have given before. Their amount of love doesn't change, they missed us. Some of us mistook their less intervention as denigrating their love. But it was not.

In the meantime, it would be a good experience if we could show the amount of love we had for our families and the people around us. It's just a wish and not a possibility. There are few things money can show but far greater what's inside the heart. Love Meter, Love Calculator, and the likes are developed, which are meant for entertainment.

There is an amount of love which never changes; it is the love of God. There might be times when I felt I was less valued, His love never changes. It is my state of mind which occupies my heart at certain times. His love never changes. It is the same forever.

As it happened, there could be times we questioned the amount of love we get. In the face of adversities, sufferings, and failures we tend to pose many questions to our God. It wasn't easy to go through such situations; our heart is filled with loneliness.

Sometimes, 'Why God? Where is your love?' could be our inner cry. We wanted to get the full love and attention of God. We wanted our adversities to be lifted; our problems get solved, in His abiding love. Yet many of the afflictions are for straightening our path although it's hard to see at the moment. (Hebrew 12:7-11)

God's love never changes, yet we missed many of them when our relationships failed. When our relationship is not good, we saw it as receiving less love.

Bargaining the amount of love we get, actually, depends on the state of our mind. When God's love never changes we took as an amount which can be changed. However, the amount towards our love for God keeps fluctuating, which causes rift inside our heart.

So in its practical sense, following God via our **dogmatically inclined practices** makes our heart vulnerable to the work of evil. Above all, God's love is the greatest and the source of all love. Any amount of love stemming out of Him could never be intolerable.

The Greatest Love of All:

When we're in love, we wanted to change the fate of our beloved in the best way possible. But since we have nothing in our hand, we can end up the other way round.

In John 3:16, the truest sense of love was found. It surpassed any amount of love in this world. The amount of love required for a man to change their life completely. The greatest amount of love was shown, given, and rewarded in giving us everlasting life.

It reads: "For God so loved the world that He gave His only begotten Son, that whoever believes in Him should not perish but have everlasting life."

This is the amount of love we get. It is always up for grab once we believe in the Son of God; Jesus Christ.

Chapter Thirteen

Fear

Fear shows its faces in our worst timing. It is two-sided; one, which decelerates our pace of thinking and living so that we have time to take care of any situations. In other words, it gives us time for second thought.

Second, fear makes the veil of hope thinner in many circumstances of life. It makes us want to build our own cocoon, if possible, trim down our passion, and unable to set certain goals in life. So, it is all powerful in both ways with huge affect o our thinking power.

Fear is abstract in nature, non-existent at times, yet can send spine chilling nervousness and pain when in action. When we are unable to tolerate it can even consume life and soul, with nothing left behind except sadness.

Here in this chapter, we would be talking about its negative effect on our living in the adversity of life. Especially for people with chronic illness, inferior, insecure, and lower background. Only one particular element can defeat fear. Keep reading whether you can agree or not.

An Old and Rusty Small Boat

One evening, two friends were late from work, on their way back home. Darkness was descending fast. All their friends reached home already. They were more tired than yesterday. But they have to cross a river on their way home.

All the boat seems to have left already. There was this old and rusty small boat, which was left for them. They are happy to have one anyway.

Someone was spying on them, they felt. Near the bush, was an old man who came forward and offers help in their situation. For the two friends, it was awesome to have a company in this situation, so they welcomed him warmly.

A second old man was approaching them, who told them he was always there in this kind of day. Now they had two old friends with them. They looked experience in whoever the field they worked.

"We don't need to introduce ourselves. Soon you will know who we are," they said. "But we are not good friends, anyway," the second old man added.

Now they boarded the old and rusty boat. The river current was stronger than yesterday.

Soon the second old man said alarmingly, "**We must go back.** We are going to get drowned, we won't make it to the other side." The two friends don't know what to do. In reality, what they heard seems good advice in their situation.

The first old man watched them patiently. He uttered, "As long as this old man is here, we won't be able to move forward. We must throw this old man in the water."

"Why?" they asked astonishingly.

"Look, young man, my name is **Faith**. His name is **Fear**." He said.

"So?"

"Fear and Faith cannot be on the same boat," he added. "And that is why we are not good friends. But we happened to exist together everywhere."

So they threw Fear in the river and strive forward to cross the river despite the strong current. They crossed the river and that is when Faith told them he did his job. So they thanked him and go their own way. hey reached home safe and sound but most importantly with a great lesson learned.

Had the first old man not win the game, they might go back or drowned in the river too. This happens many times in life. Let no fear defeat your faith in God. Have faith, pursue your goal.

Overcoming the Fear of Nothing

Future is a mystery at some level. Being a mystery instill some kind of fear in our mind. One cannot be always optimistic. That is natural. Too much focusing on the present problem may lead to unwanted thoughts.

Health problems, finance, love life are a threat sometimes. However, reflecting on the good things in the past will help at that time. There is nothing happening on us that won't benefit us. That is hard to understand, and I knew it. Here I may not be able to provide the kind of solutions you wanted but read on.

"Do not fear" was mentioned 366 times in the Bible. These are enough for the 365 days of a year. However, we failed in reminding ourselves every day about these comforting words.

I happened to came across some people who lose appetite and fear for the future among the younger generations. Just the words are empty if we failed to recognize who owned the words. Try to spend time with Him and called for external help also. Remember everyone faces that situation over different issues.

Fortune favors the brave, 'we were told. The Braves also have fear but they overcome it. When the braves failed it becomes more severe. We have to prepare for this and know how to live in the moment. Preparation may not be enough at times though. Take rest and wait for a while.

It is better to be unsuccessful than achieving our goal by any means. Remain calm. Life will take its course. The moment you become content you overcome that fear of nothing.

Wait, keep waiting, on the Lord.

Chapter Fourteen

A Safe Place: Dwelling in the Strong Tower

Avian flu, locally known as fowl plague, hit our region. We kept flocks of chicken and few ducks with us, to meet our extra demand for protein for hard-working people, and as a hobby.

It's our duty to keep them safe, as an obligated owner and protector. So, we made a hand-woven cage from bamboos to transport them into a safe place since some part of the nearby hamlet witnessed dying chickens. We do not want them to simply perish.

The news spread like wild-fire; so we act faster. Putting them in the cage, we carry them on our very shoulder as we climbed the higher mountains, where the avian flu in the lower breeze, was unable to harm them.

I can still remember carrying the very load of chicken as we try to keep them safe in the higher altitude. As according to the elders, this particular avian flu traveled with low altitude breeze for sometime in some part of the year. We did not leave them alone since we brought all our daily necessities with us, for some more time.

With a muzzle loaded gun, we watched the flocks of chicken, in the hut built on top of the hill, to keep them safe from probable attacks of foxes and hungry vixen. When it's time for feeding, we fed them with corns that we brought along. At the same time, we never kept them thirsty either.

These are the privileges enjoyed by our chickens as they have a proper owner, here it's us, as we cannot provide a safe place for all the chickens we saw. Further, some unattended chickens are more likely to bring the flu along with them should we accommodate them in the middle.

When the news of the flu leaving our residential areas was heard, we once again loaded the flocks in the cage and brought back home to release in their original surroundings. They thrived well in the place they frequented with.

It was a great joy to see them renewed life, free from the life-threatening flu which once swept the region. At the same time, it'd be a great loss on our part should we simply left them unattended to suffer from the prevailing threats of life.

It is noteworthy here that these flock of chickens cannot fly, but we walked them, carry them to a safe place, at least for a while; where they remain safe. We are a proud owner, doing good things for them, in the least.

We cannot keep the spreading flu at bay, at least for a while, but we make arrangements for our valued avian friends as we are their Owner.

A Safe Place:

Many times in our life, especially in our sufferings, we asked God to take away our pain. But God did not act at all, or we are unable to see His work, yet He kept us in a safer place. (Read Psalms 91) In His abiding grace, I'm rested in His safe place, when I needed rest!

It, really, is a great privilege for me and you to enjoy, through the blood of Christ, dwelling in the secret place of the Highest; abiding under the shadow of the Almighty. I am more than grateful I'd accepted Him as the Owner of my Soul!

I will say of the Lord, "He is my refuge and my fortress, my God, in Him, I will trust. He will cover us under his feathers. He shall give charge the angels over us; to keep us in all our ways. He made us to fly in a safer place; communing and spending time with Him.

Being our owner, our God did what is good for us. In our selfishness, we wanted Him to take away our pain and sufferings but sometimes He chose to spend time with us, in the midst of our pain. And when our strength's restored at the required level, He brought us back to live life whether it might be tough in the very beginning.

Our sufferings and pains do not consume us but could make our living hard at some level. The Lord will hide our spirit in His secret place and restore us in His time should we put our faith in Him, in stronger terms per His purpose.

Dwelling in the Strong Tower:

"The name of the Lord is a strong tower; the Righteous run into it and are safe," Proverbs 18:10 stated. In the blood of Christ, I can now dwell in the Strong Tower should I abide in Him.

I know that I'm no righteous to have the privileged of running towards Him before, but I can now run to Him, made righteous in the blood of Christ, and be safe! The Psalmist also wrote: For You have been a shelter for me, a strong tower from the enemy..... I will trust in the shelter of Your wings! (Psalms 61)

In my sufferings, there are times I almost lost hope; crushed in my thoughts as I saw no way out or I wanted an end to my pain, for my family's sake. But He whispers to me, keeping me, as I ran towards the Strong Tower of Hope.

He even let me dwell to my heart's content in His abiding grace. Like a helpless flock of chicken to make them dwell in the top of the hill so that they are safe.

"Because you have made the Lord, the Highest, your dwelling place. No evil shall befall you, nor shall any plague come near your dwelling." (Psalms 91:9,-10) The Lord is good and His words are abiding!

Abiding in Him:

In John 14:17, Jesus asked His disciples to abide in Him, so that He will abide in them too. It is important that we wanted to dwell in His words.

By dwelling in His words, we connected with Him. In the process, we are dwelling on His teachings. By dwelling in His teachings, we are dwelling in the Strong Tower, which is and set up for us.

There will be times the world would not like us, as we do not belong to the world, but by dwelling under the shadow of the Most High, He will keep us safe in His abiding grace.

The strong tower is the tower of comfort, hope, and safety even though we're still living here on earth. It is not the withering away of earthly desires and sufferings but shelter in times of need, for those who run to Him.

Our loving father, God, do not want us to perish, in the storms of life, but have eternal life. The work of evil defeated; so we have hope that our sufferings won't last forever. A new day's on the horizon. (John 3:16)

In the midst of the storm, we can meet Him in the secret place of the Most High, as we are granted access in the blood of Christ; no more or extra offerings needed for accessibility since the Spirit abided in us.

When my problems took over, it is for me to see the goodness of God and what's in store for me, although my heart tarried and memories could skip a day or two. In my helplessness, the Lord saves!

In Your Wings:

Cover me in your feathers,
Fly me; above the storms of life.
In your secret place, rest me.
Let's commune with thee.
Under the shadow of your wings,
I will abide in you.

Lead me to the Rock;
Higher than I ever could be.
Open my wings; let's flap as an entity.
Shelter my weary body,
Until it gets restored.
I run into you; keep me safe.
I need you every day.

You, who have wings,
When in need, You made me fly.
Hide me from threatening plague
I'll perish no more;
I'm glad you found me, Most High.
You are my refuge.

Chapter Fifteen

Voice of the Pilot

In the summer of 2015, with a heavy heart, I'd boarded a flight on my way back home. I was heavy-hearted because I am back from attending the funeral service of my dear elder brother's departed soul.

My mother dropped me to the local bus terminal. She reminded me to not indulge in unwanted thought and assured she'd be praying for me.

When I boarded the flight from Dimapur Airport (DMU), the pilot welcomed us. The pilot assured us of a pleasant flight in his hoarse voice. He was talking after taking a few breaks, it seems.

It was a pleasant flight until we stopped at Kolkota Airport (CCU) for allowing some passengers to join us. It rained very heavily.

In the meantime, the pilot apologizes for the delayed takeoff. After a brief wait, we take off heading towards our destination New Delhi (DEL).

Upon nearing our destination, sudden jerking of the plane can be felt inside. A likely squall from the nearby Thar Desert region seems to be causing turbulence in the plane.

We, passengers, are in panicky-mode when we are told to calm down and wait for advice from the cockpit. We waited. With the turbulence being still there, it is more than difficult to remain calm.

Passengers young and old are demanding update from the pilot in that short, long, span of time. No update was received as expected. Instead, the flight stewards are trying to calm everyone on board.

The pilot's voice might not bring good news, we don't know, but still, we wanted to hear his voice. That's when this line crossed my mind, 'the pilot who hardly speaks'.

In moments of distress, we wanted to hear some voice with authority, at least, from time to time. But the pilot did not do that. He might have his reasons but we don't know!

Then, a voice was finally heard. We are diverted to take landing in the nearby Airport available, as the condition did not improve.

We made a U-turn and headed towards Lucknow Airport (LKO), where we did refueling of the plane. There we landed.

Again, it is time to wait for the voice. Personally, with my health not in its best, it was difficult to endure such kind of journey. But I have no choice in hand.

Darkness has already descended. The four hours, the approximate, traveling time has been doubled. When we first boarded the flight we did not expect this to happen.

Again, we take off and reached our destination New Delhi airport more than five hours late. We were tired and exhausted. But finally we deboard the plane and we will be home, soon.

Now let me tell you why I narrate this journey:

It has great similarity with my own life. The usually empty heart, the unexpected turns, and U-turns. Always needing a guiding voice. The insecure heart!

In our journey of life, there is a pilot. The journey cannot and was not always pleasant. We can be empty, tired, and exhausted due to different and difficult circumstances. I am also one of them.

Many times, we wanted to hear a voice which assured us to go on even in unwanted circumstances. The voice of the pilot of our life – Jesus Christ, was unheard. Especially, when most needed.

But His voice not being heard does not mean He is not there. Yes, sometimes He remained silent. He might be silent because we did not pay heed to Him. Or, maybe, He has a far greater plan beyond we can understand.

As long as Jesus Christ is there in the cockpit, He will lead us home. He will not leave us midway.

U-turns are a possibility. Personally, when I tried to settle down the way I'd planned, I was made to take U-turn in life earning zero. But since He is there, I have hope.

Even if I did not take off from my present situation, I will meet Him one day and all my questions will be met. That voice, I longed to hear again in my journey of life.

Should there be a necessity to crash in my journey, my pilot knows what's best. I know my pilot. Did you? Will you?

One day a voice will call our name to be with Him.

Let me tell you what happen when they arrived at the Red Sea. The news came that Pharaoh had changed his mind and it spread like fire. He was coming after the Israelites with his army.

Panic set in. Pharaoh's armies were in their tail and before them was the vast Red Sea. They were thrilled at the vastness of the sea. Their sight saw no space for moving forward; they were terrified. They started blame gaming to Moses and they cried out to the Lord.

There is no road ahead for now. But the Lord said to Moses, "Tell the Israelites to move on…they will go through the sea on dry land." Moses did as the Lord commanded and they cross the sea on dry land, in short. (Ref. Exodus 14)

They moved on; they were safe. Their cries were turned into a celebration. Miriam and the women took timbrel in their hands and dance exalting the name of the Lord. (Exodus 15)

Moving Forward

Our God sometimes allows us and bring us into **"the Red Sea situation"** in our life. We cannot simply move forward from certain situations. It is beyond the wisdom of man to fathom the pain and adversities of mankind.

The vastness of the 'sea' thrilled me. I am unable to see a way out in my 'Red Sea situation'. I have no wisdom left in me that could curve a way out, even in the near future. Focusing on the intensity of my problems, sometimes, make my living very tiresome.

Yesterday I visited 'Intractable Clinic' as a follow-up, which gave me hope of me getting better with time. The reality is that such visits are a necessity for managing my health so that I could perform my daily responsibilities. It, very much, limited my role-playing in several ways needed.

I panicked easily when I encounter something un-normal when I live by my sight. When we live by sight, we act on what we can see, which is very shallow. Those projects and investments which were started with high hopes can become our 'Red Sea situation'.

I don't want to go through that pain, that brain surgery, and the after effects. But I have to move on. Move on is the advise here. The strenuous part is trying to decimate the insecure heart in submission to God.

In my journey of life, I have encountered such situations where there is no way out without God. It is He who provided water in the dry deserts, which give back life to the dry bones. He is able!

The sick and unemployed tag is something which is disheartening, but not always. I'm sorry I've revealed a lot, it seems.

Sometimes my broken brain belittles my life. It has been weakening associating with pain, from time to time. I can't take it anymore! I'm afraid to move on! I don't want to, but I have to go on. By trusting in Him, I did. And I will move on 'till I get into still waters.

The Red Sea situation turned into a celebration of the work of God. If by our mere suffering if God could get exalted; it would be worth the pain. No one will get glory except God!

Deliverance Assured:

We may cry, we may groan but His deliverance is timely and perfect. The problem is, we tend to forget the Almighty's work, even after reassuring and showing us His faithfulness.

Our God is the one who makes dry land appear out of a roaring sea. For our God, road closed sign could be an opening of a new joyful and happening era. God set the stage; He knows our needs.

Some are strained financially; some are weak physically, while some are drained emotionally. When all the aspects of life are in the doldrums, it's the real Red Sea situation. We all have our situations but our God wanted us to move on! That, we put our trust in Him; growing each day.

The devil works in innumerable ways to instill fear and discernment in our heart. But if we keep waiting on the strength of the Lord and keep moving, we will survive. If we give up on moving forward, we would be consumed. One day, when we are getting past our 'Red Sea situation' we will count the work of the Lord, in jubilation.

Once a deliverer; always a deliverer is our God! Let's move forward!

Chapter Sixteen

Don't Jump Off As Yet

It was really humiliating, that day when I jumped off a moving truck. I seldom wanted to revisit this trip as it showed the weaker side of me. Yet, I often think of it, with a smile now though.

We were sitting atop a fully loaded highway truck, which was traversing through the mountainous road. The bumpy road passes through steep walls on the other side and deep gorges on the other.

Womenfolk and children joked their way through; huge laughter ensued each time after an unraveling bump of the truck, which comforted me in a way. I was not alone, however, since it was that part of the mountain I hardly traveled, I remained awestruck through the whole journey.

As for me, I wanted to enjoy the trip in its entirety, but I'm deeply troubled inside. The truck was wobbling so hard that at one point everyone shouted out of anguish. This time, our truck was nearing falling down the deep gorge, as I saw it, and I got panicked.

When I got panicked, I don't have time for second thought. I cannot really recall what had happened in that few seconds of time.

So, I jumped off!

I jumped off the moving yet swaying truck. I found myself hanging in a small tree in the steep wall. To this day I was wondering where in the world that small tree came from. And it doesn't end there.

125

The truck did not fell through the deep gorges; it was just another wobbling-push due to the bad road condition. They waited for me once they cleared the bad stretch of the road.

It was embarrassing getting down the wall and walking down towards fellow passengers. It is one of the most embarrassing walks I could remember in my life. I simply smiled back without having the courage to look at the womenfolk.

If I could have held on for a little longer, I'd be saved from the humiliation – the Embarrassing Walk. However, the embarrassing walk can shape our perception as well.

Don't Jump Off in Your Journey:

My living has been unstable. It was wobbling; the smooth ride does come in between, yet my unlimited desire to endure the smooth ride can mislead me. I wanted the glory of God to be revealed without passing through the present sufferings.

Technically, my frail body witnessed severe wobbling, number of times, as it was seized by malfunctioning electron and neurons from the brain. The experience has never been easy for some ten years now. When our journey has been disturbed in a way beyond our control, it was sometimes hard to hold onto the faith.

We may find ourselves helpless; leading us to thoughts unlikely of certain men and women, which people couldn't digest. However, in the panicky mode of our life, and that too in longer durations, we are bound to jump off this journey called Life.

In those situations, there's one thing we should remember; the journey's not ours alone. We are only partaking with some group of people as we travel through a bit of different route set for our own good.

Don't Jump Yet: Wait Quietly

It is good to wait quietly for the salvation of the LORD. (Lam. 3:26) We might be swaying or wobbling yet slowly moving forward.

The bad and bumpy road in the mountain, surrounded by deep gorges, was a normal road for some travelers. I was just joining for a journey which lasted for seven hours. However, I jumped off as I was focusing only on the intensity of the danger moments from my point of view.

In my quest for saving myself, I could have hurt myself should there be no small tree in the rocky wall. In the road I hardly traveled, I do not know when the bad stretch will be over. However, what is more, important would be I make it to the other side. And not jump!

I could have held on to the handlebars and waited just others did. All people cared for their life, they are afraid. Some said their prayers and trust in the Lord and he comforted them.

Don't be Afraid:

There are times in life when being with good people, and the same beliefs, still evade us from true comfort. Peter was with other disciples; together they only saw the waves and the winds but their teacher. (Matthew 14:25-27)

As Jesus was approaching, they were terrified but he said, "Take heart; it is I. Do not be afraid." (v.27) Our God sees our journey through and through; he'll appear in his appropriate time should we wait for him.

Many times in my life, I draw my conclusions and jumped to my own desires where I simply ended up hurting myself. I had jumped to the deepest places not fit for a disciple to do. Yet my Savior cares for me, with which I'm saved from embarrassments.

Wherever and whenever I jumped off from His hands, the abiding Savior catches me. Unworthy and filthy I may be he always pulled me out, in his love. So, it is time for me to hold onto my little faith and that my savior gets magnified in my life.

Fear not, for I am with you; be not dismayed, for I am your God. I will strengthen you, I will help you, I will uphold you with My righteous hand. (Isaiah 41:10)

Jumping Off: Not the Solution:

I get disheartened, at times, but I don't want to. It is because there are circumstances where jumping off, is an unlikely solution. Those fear, sufferings, and difficulties will still follow us wherever we go. They would be our prize when we all get to heaven!

Paul, the apostle, had a thorn in flesh throughout his life although it was not specified as to what exactly it is. He shared what God had told him: "My grace is sufficient for you, for my strength is made perfect in weakness". (2 Cor. 12:9) In that way, there are things which needed to be endured until we're in new heaven and earth.

By trying to jump off from all hardships, or things that do not fall as we desire, we'd simply be tormenting our delicate mind. And the best part here is; people will see the face of God even in our suffering.

Now as for me, I don't know if my illness is for a lifetime, which some people often says, but it would be to endure the pain with grace.

Jumping off, although sometimes I wanted to, would lead to a greater disaster for me and my eternal soul.

Dear reader, it's better to call your friends here if you read it through, let's not jumped off while the bad stretch of our journey. We will wait on the Lord because God's works are miraculous, in the ways we cannot see. I pray He'll guide us to His purpose and desire; walking with Him closely throughout our journey.

Don't Jump Off As Yet

Don't jump off as yet
You might miss the purpose of it
Don't jump off as yet
Save yourselves from humiliation
Don't jump off as yet
You may lose out the impending joy

Don't jump off as yet
Endure your sufferings and pains
Don't jump off as yet
Although you're unfamiliar with the route
Don't jump off as yet
People are doing it too, you are not alone.

Don't jump off as yet
Wait for the Lord steadfastly
God saw your journey, He really did.
And don't regret missing out its fruit.

Chapter Seventeen

Still Small Voice

One day I drove my son to school. We were jumping topics to another; cracked up some jokes, providing the best possible answers to a number of random questions, and reviewing a few bygone years. We seem to enjoy every bit of it but we failed to acknowledge at that very moment.

We met the teacher at his school, after a brief wait, who told us a few donation opportunities. Here I won't go into the details of our meetings. Let's put it for another day or maybe not. I wanted to talk about some other things today.

My five-year-old son spent the day at school. In his brief report, he told me it went well. Now let's fast forward to our bedtime. They tucked in to get a needed night sleep. His bedtime prayer, I am so blessed to listen, every day caught my attention. It comes from him.

He thanked God for me, driving him to his school, after a short hiatus. He prayed for my good health again and again. This time it was a little different; my son prayed for my complete healing without any use of medicine.

I was on medication a long time before the birth of my son. By now, I was very much used to taking pills every day. Before I could realize, there's a problem of partial dependency on those medicines, mentally and physically.

Today, the prayer of my son instills a new hope and inspiration, that I could be free from my illness as well as shun medicines in a good way. Sometimes our much-needed encouragement from God could come through the voice of the people around us. And I am really thankful for that!

On many occasions, I'd asked my Heavenly Father to not let my sufferings and bad health, in any way, disturb the upbringing of my children. It is my hope that it would not cause them to feel inferior when they are among their friends. Rather, it could be eye-opening instances for them to witness the work of the living God.

In the Mud of Discouragement:

Let me go back a few days before this happened; I was mildly troubled by the pain and frequent dizzy spells. We missed going to church last Sunday too. It was difficult to enjoy the gatherings of people, during these few episodes.

When these episodes seized my time, it could be disheartening. It was not only me, but I also hope, who had witnessed such episodes in our life although the causal factors would vary from person to person. The causal factor could not be always health-related issues; there are many more issues which negate our happy moods.

In those moments, we could get easily discouraged. We might not be able to get out of the muddy terrain by ourselves. Nothing could help much in those situations. Going to people for help sometimes deepen the mud. In the end, people are simply people with some glorified understanding. Please note here that I am not downplaying the use of therapists and practitioners of any kind.

Now, those muddy moments could be used as a time, devoted to listening, the still small voice of our Creator; if you believe you are a created being, not some random being. In those moments, God can speak through any channel available into our heart.

Spend some time for stillness and then put it to work. I am telling you this as I've been through those muddy moments. There might be some more muddy moments, or sufferings, to come but if it is for witnessing the good side of the Lord, I won't be belligerent.

Hearing the Master's voice:

The other day, I came across Prophet Elijah fleeing for his life, as I read the Holy Bible. He was afraid of a death threat coming from Jezebel. After a day's journey from Beersheba, into the wilderness, he prayed that he might die. (1 Kings 19:1-18)

"Take my life", he said to the Lord. Although he was fed by the angels of God, he did not pay heed. He was there in the mud of discouragement. Did you notice here what he said? "Take my life I am no better than my ancestors!"

As commanded by the angel, he went to Mount Horeb where he heard the still small voice of God. In all the preceding strong winds, earthquake, and fire, the Lord was not there. But in the calmness of the place came the Lord's voice.

We do not know in what form, or through whom, voices of comfort would come. How will the Lord remind us of His presence? We can say anything about that. Anyone could be His channelized of encouragement but everyone cannot hear.

In our loneliness, helplessness, and the feeling of brokenness, for at least a moment, if we remain calm and listen we will hear our

Heavenly father speaking. He might be comforting us or may be instructing our next step.

The Rugged Road

Busy in my own thoughts I am
The road's lonely, my ride's bumpy
The rugged road's hard to tread
Jammed here in this road I chose
Silence befall, no voice I hear
Drive me out of my lonely den

My chains unshackled
In His blood I am free
Free to follow Him faithfully
Boundless love afloat my Road
Owing my loyalty to Him forevermore

Lead me in the road I'm feeble
Effete, worn, and my trembling feel
Yet You are good and faithful
Enable me to tread on heights
In fellowship, we would stay
My Rock you are my refuge!

Here in the Valley, it is dark
Pointy rocks hard to ignore
Light of hope shone my road dimly
Yet my eyes are not blinded
Your grace appeared saving me fall
Hope dawns on the rugged road!

Chapter Eighteen

Abiding Grace: Words for the Soul

Why do we study? The simple answer could be; we study so that we may gain knowledge. Employment is the byproduct of that knowledge.

All employed persons are not learned and all unemployed persons have no less knowledge either. How our learning has shaped us, as a person, is what matters.

Word by word, we learn how to read. While reading we study, which is a part of our learning. We learn to upgrade our thought, to shape our mind, and bring about change in our society, in the least.

There are words that are all-powerful; the Words of God. His words are filled with love, mercy, and grace for every soul. Powerful beyond imagination; to the saved and unsaved souls, even in their dilapidated state.

Studying Words for the Soul:

Theologians study the word of God to get a better understanding of the Words, which would eventually bring them closer to God. Yet not all theologians are filled by the Holy Spirit in their search for His fillings. It is open to one and for all.

In one bout of my Status Epilepticus; I came to witnessed how powerful His words are! In my semi-conscious state, I was told, somehow, I was uttering words, which would not have happened in my fully conscious state. And I had difficulty in recalling them.

During my ICU (Intensive Care Unit) stay, God's presence visited us in the form of His words. For some days, I was unable to have a clear thought of anything and I could hardly recall what was really happening. At that moment, hope came alive in the comfort of His words.

Several Bible verses came into my mind in time, which I told my wife or my attendants to read it out for me. Those verses came at the right time and served it right for what was most needed. Unfortunately, I am unable to recall all the verses in detail.

One after another, the verses came: the Name of the Book, Chapter, and Verses in detail. I was so 'blessed' to study the Holy Bible several times in my normal condition before I could even think this is bound to happen.

Just in time, came the verses like a flash of light. I listened to the word of God, which give me hope even in my worst physical condition. With great hope and assurance, I can sleep peacefully again and again, in His words. Some of the verses I could still remember are from; Lamentations 3:22-25, Ezekiel 37, Psalms 91 and many more.

Here I wanted to emphasize that even when our Brain does not function properly, our God has till provided His words of hope to the soul. So I am urging you to study and thrive on the Word of God, which would keep you going beyond the thought of human.

His word is a living word and He is also the living God. When flashbacks of our lives happen before us, we will need it the most. So when we have time let us read, study and learn, as the school students learned, from word to word. It will serve us good.

The word for every soul, laid bare to all of us in His flesh, during that earthly journey for a short span of time. Let us study, meditate, and learn from the Word of God – the Holy Bible. So that even in our most unwelcomed abnormal conditions, our mind might still pick up God's word from a scrap of our memories, for our comfort. Rather than studying other words, which might simply haunt us.

It's only words, some may say, but it's all-powerful. And His words will drag us closer to Him in His abiding grace.

Words; powerful enough to build a new relationship with the Almighty!

Chapter Nineteen

Whose Plan Is It Anyway?

Summer holidays for my children has just begun. I can still remember the exciting plans, which we often talked about with intense eagerness and enthusiasms, a few weeks before it finally arrived.

We were busy with their assignments and preparations for upcoming assessment in their own classes once the school reopened. Since we're joining a school we have to abide by their planners and regulations too. So we make plans together, or things to do, during their summer holidays.

First, we'd attend the wedding ceremony of our relatives. Second, we'd visit a certain number of our family friends who also visited us often. Third, we'd work on some songs of mine checking whether it fits for making their firsthand track.

Fourth, we'd visit some recreational parks or museums. And fifth, we'd watch the **Incredibles 2**, which is a 3D computer-animated superhero film and a sequel to The Incredibles, produced by Pixar Animation Studios. And many more plans…. So, we're super-excited!

I'm not writing a complete report as to how we spent the month-long holiday. But let's check out a few of them.

Deviation from Our Plan:

None of the plans were fulfilled except for the fifth one. And that too, I had to wait outside premise during the show time leaving my children almost uncomfortable.

In the first week of my children's summer holiday, I was rushed to the ER. It was an unpleasant experience, I would say, as my child had witnessed or seen what I had gone through at home or in the hospital.

There are times my caring children, aged just six and three, try walking my frail body to the washroom. They'd hold my hand in the fear that I may fall, as I sluggishly head towards the door. This unwanted and unexpected episode had affected our plans.

In my weakness, rehabilitating at home, we are unable to get out of home for most of the time. It is easy to say things more than getting done, for we do not know what tomorrow holds.

When our situation gets improved, we tell stories of the 'Faithful men of God' as recorded in the Bible. Many of life's lessons were learned by us in the process. In the meantime, when my body feels uncomfortable my children prayed for me and allowed me to take rest until we were able to finish the stories.

We even traveled back to my childhood days, as demanded by my children. A number of decades had gone by since a bunch of skinny boys, mostly underfed, wanted to be grownups.

My Plan or God's Purpose:

The Bible says, "Many are the plans in a person's heart, but it is the Lord's purpose that will prevail." (Proverbs 19:21) I feel blessed to have given the **free will** of planning my life, my activities, and beyond. But it is the will of God that will prevail.

At least for a month in my life, I cannot fulfill the plan which we laid for me and my family. We opted out for a hospital stay, as it's been a while I've been doing well health-wise. So, we opted for fun-filled summer holidays for our family and certain people around us.

Once again it is a good reminder for me, who easily rely on my meager capability and pride attitude before the Lord, that the purpose of God is always superior. In no way, I should be the one who's complaining but relying on and thanking him for every circumstance of my life.

In many ways, we struggled in accepting and understanding God's plan. If you are also one among them, like me, let's read these verses together:

"For my thoughts are not your thoughts, neither are your ways my ways, "declares the Lord. (And it simply doesn't end there) "As the heavens are higher than the earth, so are my ways higher than your ways, and my thoughts than your thoughts." (Isaiah 55:8-9 with my emphasis added)

How to Establish our Plans: (Proverbs 16)

Although I'm not good at it, I very much wanted to establish plans for my future. I, once and even now, have a plan but some of them simply did not work out, leading me in inane situations. The reasons may be many, attributing to my failure, but it is time to move on.

We have plans, we do have plans, and that's what I wanted to be reiterated here again. A person without plans is like a boat on the sea without crewmen. The boat will capsize and get lost in the vastness of the sea.

Now, the Bible taught us the right way of establishing plans: "Commit to the Lord whatever you do, and he will establish your plans." (Prov. 16:3) We must acknowledge the Lord in everything you do. Remember a smooth sailing life alone is not a successful life, but if our plans are established with God we find comfort in the unlikely situations of life too.

"In their hearts, humans plan their course, but the Lord establishes their steps." (Prov. 16:9) It's crystal clear now that it is always better to build or rebuild connections with the One who establishes our steps.

The Surprise Package – Whose Plan is it Anyway?

There was something we did which did not feature in our plan. And I believe it was there in the list, Who had planned our ways. "For I know the plans I have for you, declares the Lord, plans to prosper you and not to harm you, plans to give you hope and a future." (Jeremiah 29:11)

In the midst of our pitfall, we have this urge to spend time in the court of God. We noted down the points as we discuss and analyze our situations.

With those notes, we headed for our church which is 22 kilometers from our place. It is the first time we, as a family and only our family, spent such time in the courts of God. We give thanks, prayed, and sing: letting out our gratitude in His courts.

Our family kneeled before the Lord for me, the husband and Daddy, to get well soon if it's in the will of God. We asked for forgiveness, seeking guidance, and asking his protection for the small investments we made, and especially for our children, in the near and far future for our family.

It was worth spending every minute of it in the courts of the Lord: Our spirits lifted and our burdens lighten. This was one of the results of the troubled life we been through. It was the first time for us spending family time alone in prayer house except for the daily prayer we lead at home.

All this comes from the Lord Almighty, whose plan is wonderful, whose wisdom is magnificent. (Isaiah 28:29) It is the plan of God for our betterment!

God's Eternal Plan:

Well, without touching a bit of the biggest plan I do not want to end talking about plans. God had intended us to have eternal life; bringing us back to eternal life from the fallen world.

He wanted no one should perish but have eternal life. (John 3:16) He who believes in Him will have eternal life. Believing is living; living is non-perishing but in the realm of the eternal plan of God.

"Father, I desire that they also whom you gave me maybe with me where I am, that they may behold my glory which you have given me; for you loved me before the foundation of the world," prayed Jesus Christ for our sake. (John 17:24)

Knowing that you were not redeemed with perishable things, like silver or gold, from your futile way of life inherited from your forefathers, but with precious blood, as of a lamb unblemished and spotless, the blood of Christ. For, He was foreknown before the foundation of the world, but has appeared in these last times for the sake of you. (1 Pet. 1:18-20)

The Rewarding Plan:

Needless to say, it is hard to work out a plan which will sustain this short living here on earth. It's tougher more for me to make financial plans than before, as it takes more of brain-stretching. But I have hope that everything would be normal once again.

We wanted big houses, big cars, a good position in society, bulging or at least average balance sheet. These are the measurement of today's successes stories, which I'd lacked as of today. However, success's stories and privileged living could be another way round too.

Please remember I am not discouraging making plans or setting goals but reminding you to acknowledge God in our plans and thank Him for His eternal plan. In the end, in order that we can make a rewarding plan in our lives, we should commit ourselves to our God; acknowledging him in everything we'd planned.

The rewarding plan is the plan which acknowledges the Lord. Here I joined the Psalmist as he wrote, "Let the morning bring me word of your unfailing love, for I have put my trust in you. Show me the way I should go, for to you I entrust my life." (Psalms 148:3)

Let me end this chapter herewith Psalms 20:4,

May He give you the desire of your heart, and make all your plans succeed!

Chapter Twenty

Hold Onto What You Have

'Take it easy, hold on to what you have,' they encouraged me, 'we're here to help you.' As a young child, we're learning how to swim in the nearby river bank. For a learner, it takes tons of hard work to stay afloat in the water. When I try to swim, I sink fast, for a few days.

They, especially my elder brother and friends, sometimes my paternal uncles, assured my safety in any case. They will not let me drown, and I know that too. But when I have very few or nothing to hold on to, it was disheartening.

We don't have floatation devices in the countryside where we lived. We learn it the hard way, I would say. Sometimes we pushed each other in the water to test our ability, yet help is ever ready.

In no time, I have to master few techniques to hold on to; less I will get drown or become a laughing-stock. At least, I hold onto what I have and stay afloat, before I could swim as fast as others. It was a very wonderful experience indeed.

When in water, without any floatation devices, it requires consistent movement of our hands or leg to stay afloat. Since the viscosity of the water body is not large enough to keep us afloat, we need a few works on our part.

By the time I have something to hold onto, I could move forward to swimming although it takes courage and lots of movement of the limbs. In due course, I mastered the art of swimming. Now, just a flickering my legs can keep me stays afloat.

Should I give up before I could swim, whatever the reason it might be, I'd blew my big opportunity of enjoying swimming especially with friends. And it would be shameful as we lived in a small village near the river where almost everyone can swim.

What Do We Have To Hold OnTo?

Now, if I am to hold onto something, first, it's important to know what I have to hold on to. There should be something worthy of holding in our journey of life. While our material possession will depreciate with time, our values in the eye of our Creator stay the same.

In more than three decades of my life, I really have nothing in this material world. I possessed very little to none. What I have earned are used up in no time. Now with no job at hand, I'd accumulated no wealth. Those insurance policies I have purchased during my working days are either surrendered or discontinued.

Moreover, my health concerns me a lot. Yet I have been on to the path of recovery, I hope, which makes me happy. A little bit of broken brain but blessed to have a functioning brain; that's a privilege not all could have!

There's something more than just being healthy-wealthy and rich. Well then, there's nothing worth talking about our materialistic possession which is worth holding onto. I don't know if you agree or not.

Sometimes we have to count what we don't have, at the same time, what we lose. It is more important now, for me. This makes us appreciate what we have and value our very small or even none possession of anything viable.

Should I count them earlier, what I can really hold on to, it could have been more. But still, I am happy, for those I have lost and what I gain. I can lose some since there was a time I have some.

I have the love of my family which makes my living very beautiful. And there are these good friends I'd met and had at some point in time in my life's journey. I must hold onto them. The beauty of life is that honest and loyal people around us don't need maintenance for holding onto them.

I treasured them, yes! I don't want to lose more; less I may fumble. I wanted to hold on to them. In their love my heart finds peace; in their care, my life's needs get sustained.

With so many intrusive and influxes of unwanted or unwelcome occurrences, it is my priority to hold onto, and together, my family. If and ever I could do that with subtlety, which will require a certain amount of wisdom and intelligence with a strong fervor of love.

I shared you mine so that you can have a glimpse of what you have, in your prosperous or collapsing and depressive life. Further, I will go onto the vital feature that you and I must hold onto. Let's hold onto what we have or don't have for whom: For us, for our-self, and for our Savior.

Hold onto it until I come:

Now let's get onto what I really wanted to convey here: I really don't have anything to hold onto except for the salvation I had in Christ Jesus!

Except, for enduring some pain, poverty, and adversities there nothing much to boast about in this material world, for me. For some of you suffering souls and recovering souls, it might be the same. Although we have our own ways of suffering and withholding several tests, there's hope.

Our God had seen us. And He knows we have little strength. Yet we have to hold onto His name and not deny His holy name. We are promised to have victorious crown should we hold onto His command and endure patiently, in the name of Jesus Christ.

"I am coming soon," it was written to the Church in Philadelphia. "Hold onto what you have so that no one will take your crown." (Revelation 3:11)

We aren't demanded more; we should hold on to what we have faithfully. Holding on to His salvation we have attained through our Savior will be sufficient for securing a victorious crown. Nothing more than that! So we all have our chances, we still have something to hold on to.

"Whoever has ears, let them hear what the Spirit says to the churches," He added in His revelation to John. If not, we might have lost our victorious crown, on the way or in our journey, which is mention here.

In his first letter to the Corinthians, the Apostle Paul had stressed hard on the need to self-discipline. In other words, holding on to what we have. Here let's read: Run in such a way as to get the prize. Everyone who competes in the games goes into strict training. They do it to get a crown that will not last, but we do it to get a crown that will last forever. (1 Corinthians 9:24-27)

There is Hope in Faith:

There could be moments in our life where we feel we have nothing to hold on to. Other time, we perform our task at hand with no specific inspiration. Some of us have our 'Red Sea Situations' too. But there is hope.

It will be a good way to remind each other of the promises we have in our Savior-Jesus Christ. I'm standing on the promises of God. There is a clear implication that deliverance of the faithful will occur in conjunction with His coming.

One day we will be duly rewarded and help is on the way, soon, very soon. When our sufferings and adverse situations loom large, we might be tempted to think as if we have nothing worth to hold on to we have our Savior.

When the going gets hard to let us not lose hope. The dark night will soon get over if it's His will. For everything, there's a purpose. Let's hold on to the hope and faith we have in Jesus Christ, the Son of God.